Candid, Real Life Stories of Prostate Cancer

A COMPLETE GUIDE FOR EVERY MAN (AND WOMAN)

Dan Moore, Sr.
Adwoa Asare-Kwakye, MPH
H. Timothy Dodson, Jr.

Copyright © 2012 Midtown Urology & Marrow For Life, Inc.

All rights reserved.

ISBN-13: 978-1479205349
ISBN-10: 1479205346

DEDICATION

This book is dedicated to all the prostate cancer survivors and those who were less fortunate in their battle with the disease.

This project could not have succeeded without the help and support of all the men who participated and their candor, honesty and willingness to share their stories. First and foremost, we would like to acknowledge the ongoing support of Dr. James K. Bennett, CEO of Midtown Urology and Midtown Urology Surgical Center, who was instrumental in the design and implementation of the project.

To the people in the community who have battled or are battling cancer today, keep fighting the fight!

Dr. James K. Bennett, Adwoa Asare-Kwakye, Tim Dodson, and Dan Moore

DEDICATION

To my wonderful husband, Yeboah. Nothing in my career could have been possible without your endless sacrifice and support. You are my best friend, my confidant, and I will love you always.

To my children, Nana Adwoa and Kofi Boakye, who always greet mommy at the door with unconditional love and smiles from ear to ear even though mommy is not there to see every milestone. I love you.

To my parents, I thank you for nurturing my passion to make this world a better place and for your wisdom. To my younger siblings, Afua and Kofi, I thank you for your support and hope that you are proud of your big sister.

To my mother-in-law, Victoria, for all your love and humility, I appreciate you from the bottom of my heart and I will carry that with me my whole life.

To my sister from another, Leila, thank you for your motivation, inspiration and drive. It has helped me immensely.

To my uncles, aunts, and cousins who inspire me despite the distance, I thank you.

Lastly, to Dr. Bennett, Dr. Foote and Dr. Alphonse, the most inspirational individuals I have ever met, I thank you for inspiring me to give back.

Adwoa Asare-Kwakye

DEDICATION

To my mother, you taught me everything, and everything you've given me, I'll always keep it inside. You're the driving force in my life.

To my dad and Charles, a man has only his father to show him the way to manhood, and I've been blessed with two such figures in my life.

To Courtney, Sam, and Dominic, I hope I'm making you proud and serving as a good role model for you as you grow.

To my dearest interns, I wish you would never graduate! Monday through Friday, you are my oasis.

To BL, countless thanks for giving me a chance.

To Kappa Alpha Psi Fraternity, Inc., the Nupes have always been, and will continue to be my brothers and my support system when I need them most.

Tim Dodson

DEDICATION

Several months ago, I had the pleasure of holding in my arms, Daniel A. Moore, IV. As I reflect on this incredible experience, I could not help but appreciate the fact that had I not visited the doctor and discovered I had prostate cancer, this would not have occurred. Unfortunately, like most men if it was not broken or bleeding, the annual check-up would occur every several years.

While some of us take current warnings about prostate cancer seriously, we must now realize that the recommended age for being screened has changed. Now younger men are being admonished to test early. Early detection can make the difference in seeing your offspring or simply having them read about you in your obituary.

Dan Moore, Sr.

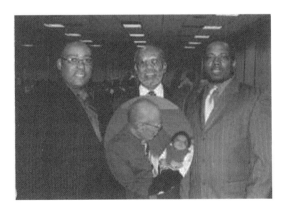

ACKNOWLEDGEMENT

To the doctors of Midtown Urology and all the people at the American Urological Association (AUA) and the National Medical Association (NMA) we would like to thank you for your continued commitment to the cause.

We would like to thank the staff, as well as interns at Midtown Urology: Briana Brown, Rachel Bien-Aime, and Ryen Smith. We would like to give a special thanks to Ariel Howard (transcriber) and Adrienne Woodall (reformatting).

Finally, we offer our sincere appreciation to our editors, Dr. Ronald Holmes and Vene Franco for their careful efforts on this tedious and time intensive task. We also like to extend our gratitude to Ms. Bev Jones and Ms. Alison Paul for our cover concept.

Dan Moore, Adwoa Asare-Kwakye, and Tim Dodson

A WORD FROM THE EDITOR

We take pride and appreciation for having the opportunity to edit this landmark book. Prostate cancer is a prevalent disease that is impacting the lives of men and their families. It is the second leading cause of cancer death among U.S. men. This book is educational, inspiring and touching.

This book allows men to courageously tell their prostate cancer survival stories and brings attention to the importance of early detection, timely medical attention, treatment selection and having the right support systems to deal with the medical, physiological and psychological impact of prostate cancer.

I am sincerely inspired by Dr. James K. Bennett's enthusiasm, passion and commitment to addressing the devastating mortality rate of African-American men diagnosed with prostate cancer. As sponsoring editor, I endorse this book as a must read for all men and specifically families that are dealing with this devastating disease.

Ronald W. Holmes, Ph.D.
Publisher and President
The Holmes Education Post, LLC
rwh@thehomeseducationpost.com
Jacksonville, Florida

The Parable of the Mustard Seed

He told them another parable: "The kingdom of heaven is like a mustard seed, which a man took and planted in his field. Though it is the smallest of all seeds, yet when it grows, it is the largest of garden plants and becomes a tree, so that the birds come and perch in its branches."

Matthew 13:31-32

New International Version (NIV)

Table of Contents

	Dedications	ii
	Acknowledgement	vi
	A word from the Editor	vii
	Foreword	xi
Chapter 1	Understanding Cancer	1
Chapter 2	The Prostate	3
Chapter 3	Stages of Prostate Cancer	5
Chapter 4	Screening	9
Chapter 5	Diagnosis	11
Chapter 6	Carrying the Torch! *Ralph Boston, Olympic Gold Medalist*	13
Chapter 7	Let Go and Let God! *Dr. George Tucker*	23
Chapter 8	We Need to Communicate! *Clayvon Croom, Jr.*	29
Chapter 9	A Family Affair! *Dr. Lamar Schell*	35
Chapter 10	The Lone Ranger! *Mr. Smith*	47

Chapter 11	I Am a Survivor! *Lee Ashby*	53
Chapter 12	Reality Check! *Clifford Pauling*	59
Chapter 13	Becoming a Champion! *Ken Stevens*	69
Chapter 14	Competing for Your Life *Curtis Lovejoy*	81
Chapter 15	The Fear Factor *Anthony Holland*	89
Chapter 16	I am not a Survivor! *Cassius Williams*	99
Chapter 17	The Check Up ***Bishop Thomas Alvin Body***	106
Chapter 18	We Have Options! *Austin Brown*	112

Midtown Urology Prostate Screening Statement	121
Glossary of Urology Terms	125
Resources	137

Foreword

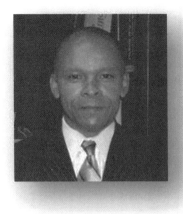

Dr. James K. Bennett, M.D., F.A.C.S

There has never been a more opportune time for a book that provides a comprehensive, intimate and candid look at one of the most prevalent, misunderstood diseases from an African-American perspective. Prostate cancer, which disproportionately strikes African-American men, has hit an all-time high in the African-American community. Unfortunately, with one in six African-American men diagnosed with prostate cancer, the raw reality of this disease has not hit home enough for many to make a lifesaving choice — a choice to educate, a choice to prevent, a choice to take charge and get ahead of what can be an extremely cruel disease.

From 1980 to 1985, I was a resident at the urology training program at Emory University School of Medicine. During this time, I first encountered this deadly disease. I noticed that it disproportionately affected African-American men, both from a morbidity and mortality standpoint. Unfortunately, very little was publicized, locally or nationally, regarding prostate cancer in the African-American community. It is from this experience that my interest grew keenly in understanding this disease and the avenues through which the African-American community could best navigate the effects of prostate cancer.

I observe men who walk through the doors of my practice every day, because they made a choice to take charge of their health. It may have been a loving wife urging her husband to be more proactive about his health; it may have been at the nudging of another persuasive family member. Whatever the motivation, the choice to pay the doctor a visit is vital. Some make that choice in the nick of time while others make it too late. Nevertheless, the choice was made. Their reluctance may be fear, pride, or simply uncertainty.

The fact of the matter is (on a public scale) the lack of knowledge, failure of leadership, and the embarrassment that oftentimes is associated with prostate cancer is preventing our community from taking a strong stance against the disease. Prostate cancer is a disease that may erode the core of a man's soul. It can affect his sense of manhood and self-esteem, and as a result, it affects his interactions with his spouse or girlfriend, and even his fellow friends. Due to misconceptions about prostate cancer, most men would rather have an affliction such as heart disease or diabetes which would be just as, if not more deadly. These fears and misconceptions are rampant in the African-American community, and we cannot, must not, allow them to continue.

It is an impossibility to defeat an enemy which is not fully understood. But given the implications of prostate cancer, many men are reluctant to openly discuss it. This leaves a huge void that comes at a very high cost. With this in mind, I took it upon myself to break through the barrier of ignorance with a powerful ideal: *actively take control of prostate cancer. This is the only way to avoid being consumed by it.* If we are to shed fear of this disease, we need those most affected to speak out about it. Hence, it is with admiration that I commend those whose chronicles have made this book a possibility. Until the silence is broken, true awareness can never be achieved.

It is from this perspective that I agreed to participate in this publication.

Enough with the mixed messages, misconceptions and misinformation! Many patients' voices have been lost throughout this controversial, misunderstood discussion about prostate cancer. It is my hope that the first-hand accounts of patients' stories in this book will plant themselves in your memory, like the mustard seed, and connect you in such a way that you, too, will be motivated to join in this fight.

Further, by sharing these stories and realizing the impact prostate cancer has had in the patients' lives, in the lives of their family, and in their community, I hope we will all be strengthened in our resolve to battle and overcome this disease. I see this book as a colossal step in bringing true light to the dire situation at hand, dispelling unsettling misconceptions, and fostering self and community empowerment. These voices are just that powerful. "Knowledge is power." And with screening, detection, and education, knowledge is life!

James K. Bennett, M.D., F.A.C.S.
CEO of Midtown Urology
Adjunct Professor, Clark Atlanta University
Adjunct Clinical Assistant Professor, Morehouse School of Medicine
Clinical Associate Professor, Emory University School of Medicine, Atlanta, GA
September 2012

"The ultimate measure of a man is not where he stands in moments of comfort and convenience, but where he stands at times of challenge and controversy."

Dr. Martin Luther King Jr.

CHAPTER 1
Understanding Cancer

What is Cancer?

Cancer is a term used to describe the abnormal growth of cells or tissue. Although there are many types of cancer, they all begin as abnormal cells and become uncontrollable.

Normal cells grow and divide in an organized fashion to create new cells as the body requires. When cells mature, they die, and new cells take their place. Unfortunately, sometimes this process doesn't always follow its course and cancer cells form when the body does not need them, and old cells do not die when they should. These additional cells are capable of forming a mass of tissue called a growth or tumor.

Not all tumors are cancerous. Tumors can be benign or malignant:

- **Benign Tumors:**

    - Are not cancerous, but can cause problems as they grow increasingly bigger and apply pressure on nearby organs and tissues.
    - Can not invade or spread to other parts of the body.
    - Normally, benign tumors can be removed and in most cases do not grow back.

- **Malignant Tumors:**

    - Are cancerous growths that have the potential to spread and cause injury or death.
    - Often can be removed, but they can grow back.
    - Cells from malignant tumors can attack and damage nearby tissues and organs.

- Cells from malignant tumors can multiply and spread to other parts of the body. Cancer cells can also spread by breaking away from the original tumor and enter the bloodstream. This can continue and invade other organs and form new tumors that can also create significant damage. The spread of cancer is called metastasis.

CHAPTER 2
The Prostate

What is the Prostate?

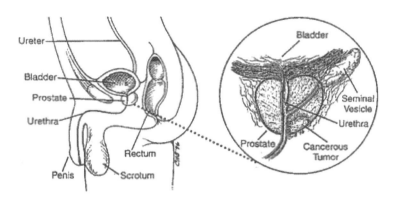

The prostate is a gland in the male reproductive system. It makes and stores *seminal fluid*, a milky fluid that nourishes sperm. This fluid is released to form part of *semen*. The prostate is located below the bladder and in front of the rectum. It surrounds the upper part of the urethra. The urethra is the tube that empties urine from the bladder.

Where is the Prostate?

The prostate is about the size of a walnut. It is located below the bladder, where urine is kept and in front of the rectum. It surrounds the upper part of the urethra; the tube that carries urine from the bladder. If the prostate grows too large, the flow of urine can be slowed or stopped.

To work properly, the prostate needs male hormones (androgens). Male hormones are responsible for male sex characteristics.

The main male hormone is testosterone, which is made mainly by the testicles. Some male hormones are produced in small amounts by the adrenal glands.

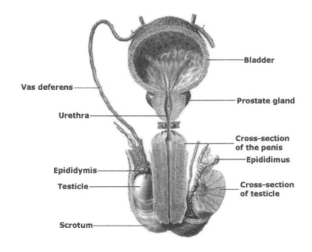

CHAPTER 3
Stages of Prostate Cancer

Following a positive diagnosis for any type of disease, especially one as deadly as prostate cancer (PCa), the first question that comes to many people's mind is: How bad is it? There are short answers and long answers to this question, but the short answers of "not that bad" or "pretty bad" do not give a complete depiction of the progression of the disease. The more you educate yourself about the disease, the easier it will be for you to comprehend and make informed decisions when selecting treatment options.

There are several ways that doctors can describe the progression of prostate cancer within the body. One very common method is the Gleason Scoring System. The other is the Staging System developed by the American Joint Committee on Cancer (AJCC).

Following a biopsy of the prostate, if cancer is found, a pathologist will assign a Gleason Grade to the pattern of cells in the tumor to classify its severity. Gleason Grades range from 1 to 5. Higher numbers indicate higher presence of abnormal tissue. The Gleason Grade of the most common tissue deformation is then added to the Gleason Grade of the second most common deformation in order to give the Gleason Score. For example, if a patient's biopsy showed Gleason Grade 3 tissue with traces of Gleason Grade 4 tissue, his or her Gleason Score would be reported as 3+4, a Gleason Score of 7. Please see Figure 1 on next page.

Cancer staging is the practice of standardizing the language of cancer diagnosis amongst physicians. By explicitly outlining the characteristics of certain phases of cancer progression, guidance for treatment can be readily developed. These staging systems typically take into account factors such as tumor location, tumor size and multiplicity, and metastasis.

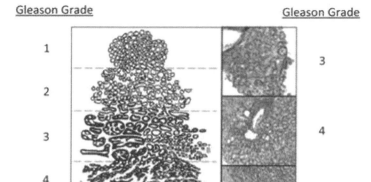

Figure 1: Illustration of tissue types as classified by Gleason Grade.[1]

The American Joint Committee on Cancer has developed several widely accepted staging systems for many different cancers, including prostate cancer. The AJCC Staging System for prostate cancer involves the clinical and pathological parameters of the primary tumor and the lymph nodes, as well as the extent of metastasis. Please see description of staging system on next page.

After a diagnosis of prostate cancer, it is always important to know what your Gleason Score and cancer staging are. These will help you to be confident in the treatment option with which you proceed. For concerns about life expectancy, consult with your trusted physician, as there is no magic formula to determine how long the disease will take to progress, if it progresses at all. Each case of prostate cancer is very unique. No charts, statistics, or search engines can replace the advisement of a doctor who knows you and your personal health.

AJCC Staging System

Clinical:

T0	No evidence of primary tumor
T1	Clinically inapparent tumor neither palpable nor visible by imaging
T1a	Tumor incidental histologic finding in 5% or less of tissue resected
T1b	Tumor incidental histologic finding in more than 5% of tissue resected
T1c	Tumor identified by needle biopsy (for example, because of elevated PSA)
T2	Tumor confined within prostate
T2a	Tumor involves one-half of one lobe or less
T2b	Tumor involves more than one-half of one lobe but not both lobes
T2c	Tumor involves both lobes
T3	Tumor extends through the prostate capsule
T3a	Extracapsular extension (unilateral or bilateral)
T3b	Tumor invades seminal vesicle(s)
T4	Tumor is fixed or invades adjacent structures other than seminal vesicles, such as external sphincter, rectum, bladder, levator muscles, and/or pelvic wall (Figure A)

Pathologic:

pT2	Organ confined
pT2a	Unilateral, one-half of one side or less
pT2b	Unilateral, involving more than one-half of side but not both sides
pT2c	Bilateral disease
pT3	Extraprostatic extension or microscopic invasion
pT3b	Seminal vesicle invasion
pT4	Invasion of rectum, levator muscles, and/or pelvic wall

Regional Lymph Nodes (N)

Clinical:

NX	Regional lymph nodes were not assessed
N0	No regional lymph node metastasis
N1	Metastasis in regional Lymph node(s)

Pathologic:

pNX	Regional nodes not sampled
pN0	No positive regional nodes
pN1	Metastases in regional node

Distant Metastasis (M)

M0	No distant metastasis
M1	Distant metastasis
M1a	Nonregional lymph node(s)
M1b	Bone(s)
M1c	Other site(s) with or without bone disease

Medical Reference

O'Dowd, Gerry J., Robert W. Veltri, M. Craig Miller, and Stephen B. Strum. "The Gleason Score: A Significant Biologic Manifestation Of Prostate Cancer Aggressiveness On Biopsy." *PCRI Insights. January 2001. Vol. 4, No. 1. Pg. 1,2.*

CHAPTER 4
Screening

What is a Digital Rectal Examination (DRE)?

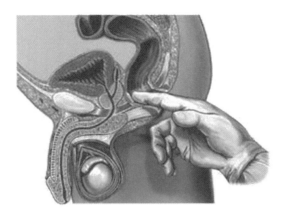

A Digital Rectal Exam should be performed annually for all men age 40 and older. This is a valuable test but it is not absolutely conclusive. When performing a DRE, because the prostate can only be reached through the rectum, the doctor inserts a lubricated, gloved finger into the rectum and feels the prostate through the rectal wall. The prostate is checked for any abnormal growths, enlargement, firmness, or roughness of the prostate. If any abnormalities of the DRE are found, the physician may order a prostate biopsy.

What is Prostate Specific Antigen Test?

The Prostate Specific Antigen blood test is used as a diagnostic tool to measure the amount of PSA in your blood. The normal PSA range is between 0 - 4.0 ng/mL. The PSA is one of the most widely used tests for detecting prostate cancer. PSA is a protein produced by cells of the prostate gland. Because the PSA can be used to detect disease, it is sometimes referred to as a biological or tumor marker. PSA levels are usually low, but can be increased due to an infection, prostate cancer and benign conditions such as inflammation of the prostate, benign prostatic hyperplasia or physical activity.

When a PSA test is performed, a small sample of blood is taken from the arm and tested. A PSA level of 4 ng/mL or below is considered normal, and a value above 4 ng/mL may be indicative of prostate cancer.

Although a PSA level of 4 ng/mL or below is considered normal, a man with a statistically normal PSA level can still have prostate cancer. The reason is that a physician is not only looking at the PSA level, but also the change in PSA level over the course of time. If a patient currently presents with a level of 1.0 ng/mL, it would appear that the patient has no cause for alarm. Nevertheless, if the patient comes to the office six months or a year later and his PSA has changed from 1.0 ng/mL to 1.35 ng/mL or above, there is some cause for alarm because his PSA velocity has increased. PSA velocity is the degree of change in annual PSA score. A man whose PSA increases by more than 0.35 ng/mL should seek consultation.

The American Urology Association recommends that a PSA test be done along with a DRE in order to determine if a biopsy of the prostrate gland is needed. In essence, men will not be able to escape "the finger" in favor of a blood test. However, PSA tests are promising in that they provide a benchmark, time-dependent assessment on the overall health of the prostate, which cannot always be monitored by yearly DREs.

CHAPTER 5
Diagnosis

If you have an exam or test result that suggests cancer, your physician will seek to determine the reason for the elevated or abnormal result. Your physician may ask to perform the following exams:

- **Transrectal ultrasound:** The physician inserts a probe into the man's rectum to check for abnormal areas. The probe sends out sound waves that people cannot hear (ultrasound). The waves bounce off the prostate. A computer uses the echoes to create a picture called a sonogram.

- **Cystoscopy:** The physician uses a thin, lighted tube (*cystoscope*) to look into the interior lining of the urethra and bladder.

- **Transrectal biopsy:** A biopsy is the removal of tissue to look for cancer cells. The physician inserts a needle through the rectum into the prostate. The physician takes small tissue samples from many areas of the prostate. Ultrasound may be used to guide the needle.

    - **If cancer is not present,** your physician may suggest medication or surgery to reduce any current symptoms you may have associated with your condition. If surgery is an option, the most common procedure would be a **transurethral resection of the prostate** (TURP or TUR). This procedure will be discussed in more detail later in the book.

    - **If cancer is present,** the pathologist will study the tissue sample from the prostate under a microscope to report the grade of the tumor. The grade tells the physician how much the tissue differs from normal prostatic tissue. It also suggests how fast the tumor is likely to progress.

CHAPTER 6
Carrying the Torch

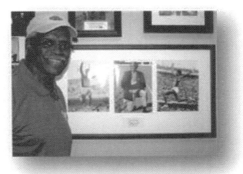

Ralph Boston, Olympic Gold Medalist

I became a patient of Dr. Bennett when I first came to Atlanta in early 2006. I had an exam, then went to the beach in St. Simons Island to have a good time. When I returned, I got a call that said, "Mr. Boston, we need to re-screen you." They did the re-screening, and my PSA was elevated a bit. From there, we started checking. I knew it was nothing I had done because I took very good care of myself. I never smoked or drank. For about 14 years, I was a strict vegetarian. It had nothing to do with my not caring for myself – it just happened.

An actor that I knew of, Cleavon Little*, died of prostate cancer. When I learned I had prostate cancer, my first thought was, well, there may be a bit of a problem. I didn't go into panic mode or anything. I just thought, let's see what comes of this. It could not be what the high PSA indicates. We did a biopsy and it was inconclusive, so we waited six months. When we did the second biopsy, they were pretty sure of what they saw. I had the procedure on Valentine's Day 2007.

Cleavon Little was an American television, film and stage actor who died of prostate cancer on October 22, 1992 in Sherman Oaks, California.

I couldn't drive for two days. The worst part about it was that I couldn't play golf for two weeks; but it was February so I didn't even play a lot of golf during that month.

The procedure I had was called seed implant. I left home about 6:15 on the morning of my procedure and was back home before noon. Other than the procedure, things have been almost the same. For me, it was kind of a no-brainer after talking with Dr. Bennett. His recommendation was, "at your stage of development, seed implant is what I recommend." Dr. Godette, the oncologist, agreed. I had to put myself in their hands because I didn't know what's best for me. I skipped med school that day!

The coach of the world famous Tigerbelles once told me a story about his getting a digital rectal exam which resulted in an inflamed or swollen prostate: Benign Prostatic Hyperplasia (BPH). It wasn't prostate cancer. His physician did a prostate massage and apparently it released the pressure from his back, and his back was no longer bothering him. His back had been bothering him prior to that point. Based on this understanding, I thought I had a back problem.

I never had a real die-in-the-woods fear of it [rectal exam]; I heard guys talk about stories – I can say it this way and I hope nobody's offended, preferably if I had to have it; I'd prefer Dr. Godette, a female physician, to do it [rectal exam]. It makes life much simpler when I leave here having heard, "you're fine." In fact, my golf game is great that day. If your preference is to have a female physician perform the digital rectal exam, go ahead and do it. The worst thing that could happen is to find out you have a problem. And if you don't have a problem, you sleep better, everything is better – even your golf game.

My doctors had my confidence because I knew them. When I first started seeing these guys, Dr. Bennett found a hernia that no one else saw. In that regard, he had gained my confidence. When I saw this guy and he said, "Okay, instead of re-treating, I'd rather just be proactive and let's go get this taken care of." In fact, I think, I remember Dr. Godette saying, "You may not have to do anything for a couple of years if you want to." My response was, "Why? Let's go ahead and get this done."

It's absolutely paramount that you believe in your physician. After all, what am I paying him for? What am I coming here for, to say, well let me think about this? I trusted Dr. Bennett.

I never told my family. Now, I'm going to tell them because they're going to read it in this book. I never told them because everything went so quickly, so well; why send them through that "Oh, God" phase, paying for flights to Atlanta and calls all night worrying about me – why send them through that?

That was five years ago, so I was 67, and at that point I don't even know what I thought. There were a couple of people who knew. One was a very dear friend that I have in Savannah. The reason that I shared that with her was that she had some breast problems. My college roommate had the problem and I never told him. He had prostate cancer and I heard his surgery was radical. But I never even told Moon; he was the track coach at Seton Hall University. We never even talked about it, other than his situation; I never mentioned to him that I had been diagnosed and was in treatment.

At some point, it's almost like I forgot about it. It was going so well until I would meet somebody who had the problem and then I would remember, "Oh yeah, I've had that." But it's almost like I forgot about it; it never happened. It happened but it never happened.

In 1997, my brother John died of lung cancer. He was 77. We thought John was in the hospital for a heart problem. We had heard, and he had made us believe, he had had some heart trouble. We didn't even know he was in the hospital. My great-nephew who worked at the hospital saw him, called his father, and his father in turn called my sister who went to the hospital and talked with the doctor. The word was then, "He won't leave this hospital alive." That was on Monday. By Wednesday, he was gone.

When I moved to this area, I invited all the family to come over and hang out. My brother didn't come. Now, I understand why he didn't come. He kept that from us so we didn't have to struggle with all of that pain. The protracted illness was there, but he never let us go through the pain of that protracted illness. For two days we knew about it, then he was gone. I remember saying at his funeral, "I hope if and when my time comes, I have the strength and bravery to do what he did so you guys don't have to worry about that." That's my story and I'm sticking to it.

When I saw that Cleavon Little died from prostate cancer, it frightened me because I had just seen him in movies and – bam – he's gone. That kind of scared me and made me think about it. But having come to see Dr. Bennett and the screenings that we had gone through, rectal exams and nothing was happening. I didn't forget about it, but it was not in the forethoughts. It was in the back of my mind as the old folks used to say.

It's not a difficult thing. If during your screening nothing is found, you're fine, go on with your life. And if it is, you can get it taken care of. In my mind, and I hope I'm right; it is not what it used to be. We have come so far with this. I remember when I first heard about prostate cancer, it was almost a death sentence. Get your affairs in order because you're out of here. Now it's different; look at me.

I have done basically the same things that I did before I had the treatment. But, I'm older so things don't happen as well as they should. I sleep a little more now than I used to sleep. I'm not as zippy or fast as I was, but I don't think my life has changed to that point.

The fact that I am still here is a miracle. The fact that I can see little Malcolm Boston II, my great grandson, and his sister Kari is a miracle. The fact that I can see my grandchildren is a miracle. But I can see now that maybe, just maybe, my standing up waving a flag, someone would say, "I know this dude, why don't I go have my prostate checked?"

First of all, and I hope this doesn't cause anybody consternation, but we're macho. We are just macho. "Ain't nothing gonna happen to me." I know that's an often used phrase – that won't happen to me. We are macho. If this makes sense, I think we are changing because I can see situations where a brother can stand somewhere and cry. When I was growing up, you would never see a Black male cry. No, I don't care if you blow off my head – I'm not going to cry. But I think I see some changes in that. The most vivid one that I remember was when we had the 1996 Olympic Games. There was Michael Johnson standing on the victory stand crying. 'Cause I know when I won, that wasn't gonna happen. And I stand there and I watch Michael in tears – whoa. So for me, I believe that's a key factor. So how do I face my buddies? I think once you realize what you've gone through and your buddies have gone through, your buddies are more amenable to say, "Hey man, welcome back." I think that's right. It feels right to me.

I'm really glad I made contact and was a patient of Dr. Bennett's, and we got this taken care of. I just think brothers should go and get tested. Go, please go! And when you find out you're okay, give me a call and let's go tee up, and I'll pay for the round.

Discussion

Throughout this chapter, the recurring message is that in this day and age, prostate cancer is not "a death sentence," as Mr. Boston so appropriately states. There are a plethora of treatment options that are available, each tailored to the specifics of the patient's age and progression of the disease. Since most men "skipped med school that day," make sure you consult with a physician **that you trust** when deciding your treatment option.

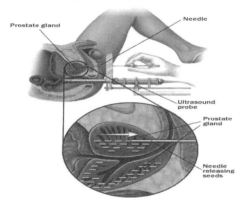

For men like Mr. Boston who have early, localized prostate cancer, radioactive seed implantation (brachytherapy) is one treatment option. You will hear this termed as "seed implants." The seeds consist of tiny radioactive capsules placed into the prostate, specifically placed for maximum effectiveness in the cancerous regions using ultrasound guidance and 3D computerized mapping.

Doctors identify the location of the tumor and map the area where the seeds will be placed. The physician then positions hollow needles to deliver, on average, 100 seeds to the prostate utilizing a special probe. Each seed is about the size of a grain of rice and remains in the prostate permanently.

The procedure is designed to provide a highly targeted dose of radiation to the prostate without harming other organs or surrounding healthy tissue. The outpatient procedure is generally done under general anesthetic, so patients typically go home immediately after treatment. Many men choose this approach as opposed to external radiation or radical prostatectomy because of the limited effect to the healthy parts of the gland. This is not to say that there are no side effects to the procedure. However, risks of urinary incontinence and erectile dysfunction can be minimized because the size of the treatment target area is reduced.

Mr. Boston also highlighted the importance of trust in your physician. Mistrust of the health care system by African-Americans is a major problem in society today. It is very important that you take a more proactive approach to your healthcare. No one is a better advocate for you than yourself.

Facts

- Brachytherapy (seed implants) is an effective treatment option with a lower risk of side effects and complications.

- Potential risk of incontinence and impotence may be reduced with seed implants.

- Radioactive seed implantation studies have demonstrated no additional risk of injury to anyone that comes in close contact with a patient who has had this procedure performed.

Recommendations

Become your own advocate:

- Speak up during your doctor's visit.
- If there is a medical term that you do not understand, ask for clarification.
- Research your doctor, the hospital, etc.
- Ask questions! Ask questions! Ask questions!
  - Who? What? Where? When? Why?

Take Charge:

- Understand your health insurance.
- Express your concerns.
- Get a second opinion.
- Ask for options.
- Find a support group for you and your family.

Medical References

Terk, Mitchell D., Brachytherapy for prostate cancer. Community Oncology. 2007; 4(2):89-92.

Kennedy, BR., et al. African Americans and their distrust of the health care system: Healthcare for diverse populations. J Cult Divers. 2007; 14(2):56-60.

Koukourakis, G., et al. Brachytherapy for prostate cancer: A systematic review. *Adv Urol.* 2009: 327945.

FACT:

"African-American Men are at a higher risk for developing prostate cancer."

CHAPTER 7
Let Go and Let God!

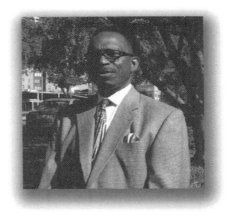

Dr. George Tucker

I am a prostate cancer survivor. I was diagnosed in 2000 and I am 11 years out. God blessed my life tremendously. I think Dr. James Bennett saved my life. Dr. Bennett was my classmate at Emory. I remember him from way back when, and he has been a true friend. God has ordained and anointed him in the areas of urology and prostate cancer. He was put here to help people: in particular, people of color and poor people with prostate cancer which is a major issue.

Some time ago, I went to Dr. Calvin McLaurin, who was my cardiologist and had my annual exams. As a part of [my] routine exam, he tested my PSA which came back as 12. I had a high PSA, so we went for biopsies. Dr. Bennett [performed] the biopsy which was positive on both sides of the prostate, so I began treatment.

Dr. Bennett and the oncologist, Dr. Eric Randolph, sat down with me to formulate a plan. I missed only two days from work during the whole treatment process that included radiation, a biopsy and prostate care. My PSA didn't fluctuate; it stayed normal. I have had very few symptoms period, and I see Dr. Bennett routinely.

About three months ago, I began to see blood in my urine. I said to myself, 'oh, snap, here we go'. So, I let go and let God be who He is, and let God do what he does. You have to do that. So, I sat on that for about a month, knowing what it could mean to me. It could mean anything, knowing what I know. Once I go in and see Dr. Bennett, the next time I come out, I could have bladder cancer. I could need a tube here; I would not be able to work and do this thing that God has anointed me to do anymore. It could be life changing. Just tomorrow, if I go and see Dr. Bennett, my life could change. I may not be able to provide for the family anymore; who knows? So, I thought on that for a minute. Finally, I did the right thing. I talked to my oldest son who is 40 – he's a physician, an OB/GYN. Rightfully, he told me, what I already knew, to get it checked.

The first defense mechanism that people have is denial. We think "that ain't me – I don't have that – I ain't got cancer, he has this all wrong." You say, maybe it ain't my biopsy – denial, denial, denial.

And then the reality sets in when all the pieces are in place. I came in and Dr. Bennett said, "George, you need a cysto." I had a cystoscopy and it was negative. I had a CT scan (computerized tomography) of the kidneys and it was negative. Then I had some peace that everything was good. My mom taught me – she's such an angel – that everything in life is ordered by God. I found peace and solace in that and that carries me.

I don't ever get up in the morning thinking about cancer. I ask God each day to give me somebody's life I can walk into and make a difference. This is my 30th year of practice and I find myself with the resources and the ability to help people. What a sin it is to have a gift and not share it.

I often ask myself, what has my prostate cancer done for me? First, it brought my family closer together. I also realize that if I have a genetic disposition, I can tell my boys and this can help them. My story could've been different if Dr. Bennett hadn't been in my life. And throughout the process, I did not always have insurance. It didn't matter to Dr. Bennett; he was my friend and he worked with me. Dr. Bennett said, "We'll work it out." He has been an anchor in the management of my health care.

As for Black men, we have a horrible problem going to the doctor even if it could be life changing. It's part of being a man, it's part of what we do. We don't expose ourselves. We don't show weak spots. We don't show things that hurt a lot. We hide things. We hide how we feel about the wife or the relationship with the child. It's the nature of men – We always keep stuff inside – And some of it is cultural – It's a man thing. I guess, men see themselves as less in terms of sexual prowess and in terms of sexual ability, in terms of being that guy.

I think, a man thinks it diminishes him. What he has to come to realize is that there are other parts in life: there's the wife, the grandkids and other important people in your life. From about age 30, men lose about 2% of their testosterone a year. At 40, there's no problem. At 50 and 60, it's a problem. It's just part of the process of aging. Just like your muscles get weak and your hair goes away. It's just part of getting old – this thing will sneak up on you.

The question often arises about the disparity in health care. We as Blacks have more to deal with than anybody. If I go to the hospital, I don't always have access. If I go to a hospital and they treat me like I'm a roach, like I'm nobody, I ain't going. So access isn't always access. If I go to the hospital and I'm made to sit 10 hours and you talk to me any kind of way, I ain't going. The cost of medical care limits us. If I go to the hospital and I don't have insurance or a job, I can't get a sliding pay card; I just have to live with the disease.

Discussion

Dr. Tucker mentions an issue that is ever-present in the male mindset: an unwillingness to acknowledge health problems. In many of our testimonies, there is a very common theme that replays itself. From a young age, girls are coddled when in despair. Whereas, boys are taught to "suck it up," "stop being a girl" and "walk it off." This mentality is refined throughout adolescence and into manhood, such that it becomes acceptable for men to bear pain.

Athletes play hurt so as not to abandon their teammates. Fathers trudge to work in pain to provide for their families. Their endurance is valiant, but where should the line be drawn? There is a significant difference between a knee scrape and painful urination. The sad truth is that many men see no difference.

Fear of knowing is intimidating. People, not just men, tend to live by the principle, "ignorance is bliss." The mere implications of a prostate cancer diagnosis are detrimental to the psyche of the patient and to the morale of his family. It is acceptable to consider the ramifications of knowledge and its inherent psychological effects.

For example, patients suspected of carrying the gene for Huntington's disease, a neurodegenerative condition that leads to dementia, sometimes choose to forego their option to be tested for the genetic defect in the hopes they can maintain peace of mind. However, it is not acceptable to ignore the consequences of succumbing to a *manageable* disease, like prostate cancer.

Awareness of prostate cancer can only account for some of the increase in early diagnosis that we would hope to see. Our communities must change our culture and thinking about the importance of early detection and care.

It must be noted that Dr. Tucker actually found a positive influence created by his diagnosis. His condition strengthened the bond with his wife and allowed him to educate his children, such that their knowledge could serve their own benefit.

It is important that men with prostate cancer envelop themselves in a sense of conscious optimism. In doing so, admission of vulnerability may cease to be as taboo. The world is too progressive for men to have closeted sentiments about their physical health and overall well-being. By teaching our boys to express themselves appropriately, we will eventually have a generation of men willing to speak out about their health conditions. This is the only true means to breaking the silence.

Medical References

Lee, DJ., et al. Barriers and facilitators to digital rectal examination screening among African-American and African-Caribbean men. Urology. 2011 Apr; 77(4):891-8.

Wagner, SE., et al. Cancer mortality-to-incidence ratios in Georgia: Describing racial cancer disparities and potential geographic determinants. Cancer. 2012 Jan 31. doi: 10.1002/cncr.26728.

CHAPTER 8
We Need to Communicate!

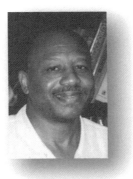

Mr. Clayvon Croom

I'm originally from South Carolina. I attended Cheney State University in Pennsylvania, came to Atlanta University in 1978 and received a Master of Business Administration (MBA). I have a pretty large family; there were 14 of us. We were basically farmers. My dad was a veteran of the military; he died of prostate cancer in 1990. He called and told me about the prostate cancer. He knew he had it, but it was one of those things he thought it would go away. By the time the news reached me, it had moved to his bones.

I knew Dr. Bennett from school. We attended Atlanta University together. I brought my dad to Atlanta to see Dr. Bennett. Howard University was doing research on prostate cancer and its possible genetic connections. They drew blood from my aunts and uncles for research. We discovered that all my uncles had prostate cancer – in fact, seven of them, including my dad. My dad was the first to die from prostate cancer and his oldest brother was next. A couple of my uncles are still living with prostate cancer because of the medical developments from the time my dad had it until my diagnosis in 2004. Prostate cancer is something I've been watching and Dr. Bennett's been following me since 1992.

I've been getting checked every year since 1991. Because my PSA jumped from 1.8 to 2.4, there was concern. I came to see Dr. Bennett actually thinking nothing was wrong. He advised that, because I had such a family history, he needed to perform a biopsy. I received the results upon my return from a business trip. I was expecting to hear, 'well it was negative, everything's fine.' When Dr. Bennett walked in, he looked at me funny and I knew something was wrong. He broke the news to me and told me my situation. It shook me for about an hour. I recall very vividly when I was told I had prostate cancer, my very first thought was, 'How long am I going be here?' The only thing I was thinking about was how many years I had left and what I need to do. I was told the average lifespan of a Black man living in Atlanta at the time was 61 or 62. I said, "Well, I need to leave and go back to South Carolina!"

I reverted to my knowledge of the disease. I made a decision years before, if I get prostate cancer, I'm going to have it removed. At the time, I had a four-year-old and a six-year-old, and I needed to be around. I can't get caught up in anything else. That next day, I called Dr. Bennett to schedule my surgery. He said, "You need to have some time to think about it." But, I'd already thought about it. I couldn't think any further than this. Dr. Bennett performed the surgery, and I've had absolutely no problems so far. I thank God for that. Erection? No problem.

We need to put the biggest face we can to the cause. We've got Black churches. We've got Black athletes everywhere ... It has to be communicated. We have Black colleges; communicate it. We have Black organizations that are strong; send a message. But we prefer to talk about a whole lot of things rather than the things that are most important to us and to our survival. I ran into a slew of guys coming into Dr. Bennett's office who were battling prostate cancer at the same time that I had prostate cancer. They would never tell anybody. Sealed lips and the refusal to spread the word is a brand killer. It's a branding killer. You can't brand a disease if people won't talk about it. You must open up and let the world know that this thing exists.

I've had conversations with a number of guys because I'm on the patient advocate list. We consult with the guys who are recently diagnosed. The biggest concern I see with Black men is about sex. What happens to them sexually? For me, I have some young sons, and I want to spend some time with them. I want to see them grow up and become men. I wasn't caught up in the sexual thing. Although things turned out very well for me, I consider myself lucky. Erection comes to me like plucking your finger. I never used Viagra or anything like that. So I've had good results from it. A good buddy of mine said, "Man, why you go and do that? You're going to end up with something to just pee out of." I said, 'Well, I don't know about that, but as long as I'm alive to pee, I'm happy.'

I've had a lot of guys call me and thank me for getting tested and treated early. Otherwise, they would have been sitting back waiting. And waiting is not a good thing. I explained that to these guys, "Listen, you don't have that luxury because there are some guys that we know passed on, a lot of them at my age and younger." Whenever they call me, they get the real story.

One of my friends had prostate cancer and it slipped outside his prostate. He had to go through a series of radiation treatments. I often called him and I would always ride him about getting checked because we are the same age. He comes to me now and says, "Clay, you saved my life." Early detection is everything. For me, I had no bad experience with it. I am here to see my family grow up and to simply enjoy life. Man, if these guys only knew that.

Discussion

Radical prostatectomy is one of many ways to combat prostate cancer. It is a surgical procedure that completely removes the prostate gland and some of the neighboring glands and tissue. It offers an opportunity for long-term survival to patients whose cancer has remained localized within their prostate. This way of treating prostate cancer is generally effective in those patients who have been fortunate to have the cancer contained within the prostate.

Mr. Croom had an extensive family history with the disease; from the time of his father's diagnosis 14 years prior until his own. He had been preparing himself for the choice that lay ahead. For him, the decision was made long in advance. To those who are blindsided by their diagnoses, consult with **a trusted physician** to make sure radical prostatectomy is the perfect choice for you.

Facts

- Open Prostatectomy
    - **Retropubic -** The surgeon creates a cut through the abdomen. Perineal is the method.

    - **Perineal -** An incision in the area between the testicles and the back passage.

- Laparoscopic Prostatectomy
    - **Keyhole prostatectomy** - The surgeon creates an incision in the belly of the patient and then inserts a viewing instrument called the laparoscope into one of the incisions to guide removal.

    - Robotic surgery is also performed laparoscopically.

- Most men who go through with radical prostatectomy often deal with erectile dysfunction (ED) and urinary incontinence to some degree as post-surgery problems. These disadvantages vary based on the age, health and stage of cancer of the men undergoing the surgery.

- Patients will be required to remain in the hospital for approximately 2-4 days; a catheter will remain in the bladder to drain the urine for 1-3 weeks.

- Radical Prostatectomy is not an option for patients with metastatic prostate cancer.

Recommendations

- Consult with **a trusted physician** to make sure radical prostatectomy is the perfect choice for you.

Medical References

Lepor H. Open versus laparoscopic radical prostatectomy. *Rev Urol.* 2005; 7:115–127.

Marks, Sheldon. Radical Prostatectomy – A Surgical Solution. Prostate & Cancer: A Family Guide to Diagnosis, Treatment & Survival. Tucson, AZ: Fisher, 1999. 157-95.

Radical Prostatectomy. WebMD - Better Information. Better Health. 21 June 2010. Web. 01 Aug. 2011. <www.webmd.com/prostate-cancer/radical-prostatectomy-operation>.

CHAPTER 9
A Family Affair

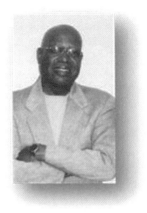

Dr. Lamar Schell

I was born in Atlanta, Georgia in Vine City on the west side and went to Turner High school which is currently closed. I am what is known in Atlanta as a Grady Baby because I was born in Grady Hospital.

I am the youngest of four brothers. The brother who I am closest to is James. There is a 12-year difference between the two of us. My oldest brother is Luther, and he is 17 years older than I am. My second oldest brother is Anthony. My father and brothers put their money together and built a brick, two story house with a basement in the 1940's.

When I graduated from high school, I did not have any money to go to college, so I worked for a year at Grady Hospital. Afterward, I went to school at Albany State University where I received an undergraduate degree in biology with a minor in chemistry. I went to Georgia State University and received a master's in Science

Education. I also went to Atlanta University and received a doctorate in education. I taught for four years in Fayette County, but I spent most of my career in administration.

The first year that I taught was the first year of integration in Fayette County. It was odd because all of the African-American kids would gravitate towards me while the Caucasian kids would stay at a distance. It was a school that had been condemned, but Fayette County needed the space so the county reopened it. In about two or three weeks, everyone got comfortable and came together. It was an incredible experience. It was just so stimulating for me to see the students learn and their eyes light up when I taught them something new. In 1997, I retired as an elementary school principal.

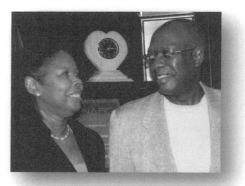

Dr. Schell & wife Yvonne Schell, M.Ed.

I met my wife, Yvonne, when we were taking an English class at Albany State University. She had long hair and looked incredible. She told me that she lived in Dawson, Georgia, 25 miles away from Albany, Georgia. I did not have a car, so I could not go to Dawson. The next year when I saw her, I asked if she was still living in Dawson. At that time, she was staying in town, so we started dating. She graduated before I did. When I graduated the next year on a Saturday, we had our wedding on a Sunday. We came back to Atlanta and lived at my mother's house until we got our own place the following year.

I asked my brother, James, if he could recommend a doctor because I was having urinary problems. He recommended Dr. Bennett. I would feel a great urge to urinate often while driving. It was so uncomfortable that I would have to pull over before I reached my destination; I just couldn't wait. I trusted my brother's recommendation and sought the opinion of Dr. Bennett.

After my exam, I was told my symptoms were related to my prostate. Dr. Bennett diagnosed my condition as an enlarged prostate (benign prostatic hyperplasia or BPH). He recommended sending an instrument through my urethra to remove the section of the prostate that was blocking my urine flow. It worked wonders. Dr. Bennett told me that he would also take samples of the tissue to see if the prostate was cancerous. Urination was no longer a problem. However, cancer was found in my prostate. Dr. Bennett carefully went through all the alternative treatments. I then talked to my loving wife. We both felt that it was best to just remove the prostate and be done with it. I chose the radical prostatectomy; the complete removal of my prostate. I was fortunate that I came early, so Dr. Bennett was able to contain it in the prostate. At my age of 52 and with my family history, there was no doubt in my mind what needed to be done.

Anthony, my second oldest brother died of cancer in 1973 at the age of 44. In 1973, our family knew very little about prostate cancer, so we do not know the origin of his cancer. My brother James died in 1999 at the age of 67. All of my brothers had cancer, so I was not too optimistic about this. My brother Luther had someone else perform his operation before he came to Dr. Bennett. He did not come to Dr. Bennett until after it spread to other organs.

When I think about the procedure, I guess I was never fearful because of my science background. Some of it was interesting to me! I always said, "If you weighed one against the other, you have two choices: life or death." I once said in a paper I wrote, "It was just so much I would have missed if I had decided, no, I'm not going to do that only because I had reservations about rectal examinations.' I had a friend who was like that, and he is no longer with us because he waited too late. He would always mention to me that, "Nobody is going to put that thing in my rectum." But when you think about it, you should know what you are risking. Life is valuable not only for me, but also for my family. It is important to them for me to be here. After the surgery, I realized that I was going to survive. I started thinking about how valuable life is. I started thinking about the small things that I did not think about before. I think that has made me a happier person. I don't worry. My wife Yvonne says that I am not as grumpy as I used to be.

My wife, Yvonne, played a very significant role in all of this. We are retired now and are having more fun than we ever had. We have time for each other now! During my journey with prostate cancer, it was always Yvonne's concern more than anything that I stay alive. She wants me to be with her more than anything else in our retirement.

She is a very calm and rational person. It is easy to talk with her and we do not hide things from each other. She created a comfortable situation. We have been able to work together and do many things that many people our age cannot do. Her support has been paramount. I have never felt that I had to make the big decisions alone. We could sit down and talk. That has been really important.

I think a wife should be informed, supportive and understanding. She should come to conferences and learn about the disease. Yvonne has always said that she just wanted me to survive. She goes to all of my checkups with me. She knows exactly what is going on with me firsthand. Sometimes it makes doctors nervous having her in the exam room, but I need the support. I think that the doctors got used to it after a while. I do not keep things from her; she knows exactly what I know. The irony in it is that I tried to go in with her on her exams, but understandably her doctor would not let me in, so I had to wait outside.

Now when we get into the sexual aspect of prostate cancer, of course, that is a major problem with many people, especially me. I went through all of the things that I could use such as Viagra and other pills. The problem with Viagra was that it seemed to raise my blood pressure. I could feel my heart racing. Yvonne would put her hand on my chest and she could feel the tension. It bothered her quite a bit. They had a mousse, a suppository you put up your urethra, and an injection that is placed into the penis. None of that went well for me. Consequently, we finally settled on the Osbon Vacuum Device. It works well for us because it always works. We worked all of that out and now we have a very satisfying sex life. I really appreciate the understanding Yvonne has given. She made sure that I did not worry about anything. We worked things out quite well.

Now at age 67, 14 years later, I am free of the cancer. It has been great! I guess I was fortunate that I watched my brothers and saw how our physiology was quite similar. When they started having problems, I suspected it was going to happen to me. I did not think it would be that similar. I thought I would be in my sixties before anything happened to me. It would not have been good for me to just wait and wonder, so now I am free of it. Yvonne and I are both very happy about our decision for me to have surgery.

My son feels that as long as I'm fine, he's fine. He didn't like the breakfasts I was eating with the bacon and stuff, but he didn't say much about it. What he did do was make me breakfast on the weekend. He would get up around 6 o'clock in the morning and begin cooking before I could cook. He'd measure how much eggs and bacon I got, if I got bacon. If he made pancakes, I'd have to slip downstairs and get some more syrup because he never put enough syrup on the pancakes – you know, cutting my calories – he's a real character.

My son checks on my health all the time. Even when he was a little kid, he was like that. When I went in for surgery, he went berserk. He was about 10 years old and took my condition very seriously. He doesn't take my illnesses well. Even today, he is like that. He adjusted the level on our treadmill so that I would work a little harder. That's the way he thinks. He'll make suggestions. He's got me eating oatmeal instead of fried foods and he is really concerned about my cholesterol. So, it was a thing where I needed to be here for him to be able to go into adulthood, and I wanted to be here for my wife also. It just worked out so well for me.

Now, it's my responsibility to talk to my son about getting tested. He's 30 now. Since cancer is so prevalent in my family, it's best for him to start getting checked for it now. And my advice to any person is that once you get in your late 30's or 40's, especially African-Americans to get your prostate checked. Things have advanced more since I had prostate cancer. If the cancer is detected in time, there are now more viable options to make informed decisions about your care.

My advice to men, especially Black men is: Don't let yourself get caught up in taboos and superstition. This extreme masculine mentality can be deadly. That's the problem, it can actually be deadly. You just have to weigh one against the other: life or death. That's pretty much it – that's the critical thing to think about. But, I've got friends who told me about relatives who said, "No, no, I'm not going to have a rectal examination," and they died from it. To die because of ignorance is a terrible price to pay, especially when there are so many options that people have now.

I was talking to a friend of mine and he was telling me that a buddy of his has a pump, and his girlfriend asked, "Did you bring the pump?" So, people can adjust to things. Humans are extremely good at adjusting, and I think with that thought in mind, you can adjust to almost anything.

Discussion

There are three main themes in Dr. Schell's story that are important to discuss:

- Hereditary Prostate Cancer (HPC)
- Benign Prostatic Hyperplasia
- Role of women and family in the awareness of prostate cancer

The specific causes of prostate cancer are unknown; however, research has shown that men are predisposed to prostate cancer based on certain risk factors, e.g. age, race and family medical history. A risk factor is something that may increase the chance of developing a disease.

Dr. Schell's family history of prostate cancer provided him a warning of his condition. Research has shown that a man's risk for developing prostate cancer is one and a half to three times more likely if his father or brother is diagnosed with prostate cancer than if he had no family history of the disease. In Dr. Schell's case, he had three brothers diagnosed with prostate cancer. The likeliness that Dr. Schell would get cancer during his lifetime was significantly increased due to his family history. As a result, it was imperative that Dr. Schell get screened due to his increased risk for prostate cancer attributable to his family history. The table on the following page illustrates an estimate of how these factors affect risk. It details how a person's risk increases with the number of relatives affected with prostate cancer.

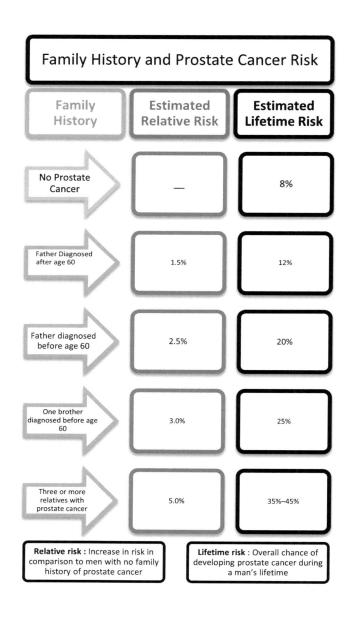

Table 1: Source: Bratt, O., J Urol 2002; 168:90.

Benign Prostatic Hyperplasia (BPH) is another condition described by Dr. Lamar Schell. It is one of the most common problems affecting men over 50 years of age.

According to the National Institutes of Health, the estimated prevalence of BPH is 24% for men age 40 to 49, 31% for men age 50 to 59, 36% for men age 60 to 69 and 44% for men age 70 or older.

BPH is a non-cancerous enlargement of the prostate that usually causes difficulty with urination. The prostate "squeezes" the urethra as urine is voided, making this process more painful. The most common symptoms of BPH include:

- Getting up at night to go to the bathroom
- Difficulty starting urine stream
- Sudden urge to urinate
- A weak urine stream
- Painful urination

These symptoms suggest BPH, but they also can signal other or more serious conditions. BPH is NOT a form of prostate cancer nor is it a risk factor for prostate cancer.

Every year, approximately 14 of the 19 million men with symptomatic Benign Prostatic Hyperplasia (BPH) go undiagnosed. The following chart speaks volumes to the extent of how this condition affects the average male.

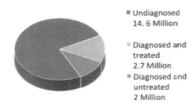

More than 14.6 million men go undiagnosed with this condition. As a result, it is very important to tell your doctor about any urinary problems that you may have such as those described above. As previously discussed, BPH is a condition that commonly causes lower urinary tract signs and symptoms (LUTS) such as weak urine stream, incomplete emptying, increased frequency, urgency, weak force of stream, etc. These signs and symptoms are related to compression from the enlarged prostate to the urethra. It is very common for the prostate gland to become enlarged as a man ages. As the prostate enlarges, it compresses and distorts that part of the urethra which passes through it, causing disruption to the normal flow of urine similar to a clamp on a hose.

Women influence their spouses' experiences of prostate cancer, and they are also significantly affected by living with partners who have prostate cancer. As such, prostate cancer has emerged as a "couple's illness."

Patients should be encouraged to bring their wives or loved one with them during their visits and follow-up appointments. The rationale is that many times, physicians would repeatedly ask their male patients, "Do you have to get up during the night to void?" They would respond no. On the other hand, their wives would respond and remind their spouses that they got up at 10:00 p.m., 12:30 a.m., etc. to void. These things are very important for a physician to know which can assist in the overall diagnosis of your condition. Also, the information you provide the physician will give the entire picture of your current symptoms.

Facts

- 14.6 million men with symptomatic BPH go undiagnosed.

- A family history of prostate cancer is an indication that you are more likely to develop prostate cancer, apart from the fact that African-American men are more at risk of prostate cancer.

Recommendations

- Research your family history regarding prostate cancer.

- Because hereditary prostate carcinoma is characterized by an early age at onset, first-degree relatives in high risk families should begin screening before age 50.

- Be sure to monitor your benign prostatic hyperplasia by getting your digital rectal exam and prostate specific antigen tests yearly.

- Take the time to include your loved one or partner in the decisions. Bring your loved one with you to talk with the physicians during your clinic visits. Let your loved one know that their contribution is important.

Medical Reference

Boehmer, U., Clark, JA. Married couples' perspectives on prostate cancer diagnosis and treatment decision-making. Psycho-Oncology. 2001; 10(2): 147–55. 39.

CHAPTER 10
The Lone Ranger

Mr. Smith, Prostate Cancer Patient

I'm from a little town called Helen in West Virginia. My father was a coal miner. I left and went to the Marine Corps. I stayed in the Marine Corps for four years, did a little traveling and later moved to Michigan. I worked in the steel mill in Michigan for 13 years. I never liked the mill or Michigan. However, it afforded me the opportunity to read occasionally. I started reading about some things, and looked at where I thought I'd go if I stayed at that steel mill – nowhere.

I decided to start making some changes in my life by moving either to Florida, Texas or Georgia. I did a little research and started reading *Ebony* magazine, particularly about a contractor named Herman Russell. From this, I decided to relocate to Georgia. I moved to Atlanta in 1978. Although I had never been to Atlanta, I came on a Sunday, got into real estate school on Monday and I've been here ever since. And I love it.

I first started to notice problems with my prostate after having sex. It was hard to urinate. I had no idea what a prostate was. I had just come out the military and went to the Veterans (VA) Hospital when the doctor told me it was infected. The doctor gave me some antibiotics that took care of it and I went back to doing my normal things. It didn't affect me until I turned 40. A young man at the VA told me, "You need to start taking care of your prostate because in Black men, it can cause some serious problems." At that time, I didn't hear him. I was a young dude, and I was running around having a good time. We call it, 'the ditch,' out in the street. I said, 'Well, whatever they're talking about, it's not going to affect me." So

I rocked on like that another six to ten years. Finally, I noticed that my prostate had gotten to the point where it was hard for me to urinate. I went back to the doctor and he gave me more antibiotics and it would be okay.

At that time, I did not know the seriousness of what could happen. I hadn't known anyone who experienced cancer, so I didn't know what to expect, which in hindsight was to my benefit. I never thought that I wanted the prostate taken out. I didn't know what it did. I didn't know what function the gland performed. I never thought about removing the prostate until I learned about the alternative options.

After I came to Atlanta, somebody told me about Dr. Bennett. He's been my doctor for over 20 years. He would check my PSA, tell me to watch my diet and the like. As I got older, I started reading stuff, watching what I ate and doing a little exercise. Ten years ago, I was diagnosed with prostate cancer. The treatment we used to address my cancer was cryotherapy (cryo). Eight years went by and the prostate cancer flared up this past March. But now, I'm okay.

The first time I did the treatment, it wasn't that difficult. After the second cryo, it's a little more so. Sometimes I get a weaker erection; I'm told this is normal after some of the nerves are damaged. The positive thing is, I still get an erection. That was one of my concerns from the beginning, and it's not hard talking about it. But, this is the first time in almost 10 years that I have talked about it.

It has been ten years since I was diagnosed at age 59. Before I started seeing Dr. Bennett, the only time I went to the doctor was when I had trouble urinating after sex. After they gave me the antibiotic to fix the problem, I'd go back to doing what I normally did. Before the diagnosis, I always loved life. I didn't really think about prostate cancer before the diagnosis. I would think it's not going to happen to me or I didn't think of the seriousness of it. And, I don't know if I consciously watched my diet. I do remember reading about the Nation of Islam which stopped me from eating red meat and pork. I was coming to the realization that I needed to start taking better care of my body.

I never felt that the cancer was life-threatening. I was never really scared. You try to change some of your habits – you come to realize or learn what's important such as trying to take some preventative measures. But, I never really felt threatened.

Now, I'm thinking that when I got diagnosed with cancer, it changed a little bit. I started looking at some of the other things that I could do to cut the risk or keep the cancer from recurring. A lot of the things that I was eating before, I didn't know affected me, like fatty stuff. I didn't eat a lot of fried foods, and I didn't drink as much. I never smoked. So, I think I started having sex a little bit more.

It's sad for me to tell you, but I have four children and to this day, they don't know about my prostate condition. This is not an excuse. I think the decision I made, is a valid one. The same day that I was diagnosed with cancer, my ex-wife had a stroke and my oldest daughter found her the next morning on her way to work – this was her second stroke. I made a decision that my children didn't need to try to digest all of that at one time. I didn't tell them and until this day, I still have not told them. My ex-wife died not long after. I saw the effect that it had on my oldest daughter. Rather than unloading my prostate condition on them, I sheltered them. I didn't discuss it because my condition wasn't life-threatening. Less than a month ago, I saw my daughter and she had a defibrillator, gastric bypass surgery, and a pacemaker put in. One of the things she mentioned to me while I was there was, "I got enough on me, you don't need to die on me anytime soon."

Only three people know about my condition; the woman I was dating, my brother, and a guy I work with. Those three people know – and you, now. I haven't told my 46 year old son because our relationship is kind of sorry. He wanted to know why I didn't visit his mother after her second stroke. The reason was, I got the news about my cancer on the same day they [the children] called me about her stroke.

I've got to get involved in some meaningful way to support cancer awareness. I've been trying to figure out how to do that. My son is here in the city, and I have indirectly sent him Dr. Bennett's card with a note telling him that he needs to get his prostate tested. I don't like people wanting to know if I'm okay when they see me. Sharing my experience in this book is helping me to figure out how I can get involved some kind of way. 'Cause, I'm going to get involved; I just don't know how.

Discussion

Mr. Smith, like our other featured interviews, represents an African-American man that was affected by prostate cancer. As we have learned by now, the Black community is disproportionately affected by this disease. We have related the incidence of genetics, but there is nothing we can do to change our genetics. We must focus on the things that we can change: awareness, knowledge and action.

The only way to change trends in large populations of people is changing their culture and mindset. We do not have the power to change genetics and ancestry, but what we can change is the knowledge gap in our communities. To date, there has been no successful campaign to educate the general public on the epidemic of prostate cancer in **any** community, much less that of African-Americans. This has to change.

Facts

- Incidence of prostate cancer in African-American men is 58% higher than in their white counterparts which is the group with the next highest incidence.

- Death rates from prostate cancer in African-American men are more than two times those of their white counterparts, and more than **three** times that of other races.

Prostate Cancer Statistics		
Racial/Ethnic Group	Incidence	Death
All	168.0	27.9
African-American/Black	**255.5**	**62.3**
Asian/Pacific Islander	96.5	11.3
Hispanic/Latino	140.8	21.2
American Indian/Alaska Native	68.2	21.5
White	161.4	25.6

Statistics are for 2000-2004, age-adjusted to the 2000 U.S. standard million population, and represents the number of new cases of invasive cancer and deaths per year, per 100,000 men.

- According to Us TOO, a prostate cancer awareness organization, there is a 19% chance (1 in 5) of being diagnosed with prostate cancer and a 5% chance (1 in 20) of dying from it.

Suggestions

- Spread your knowledge of prostate cancer and prostate cancer screenings to the men that you know: your sons, brothers, fathers, grandfathers and uncles.

- Encourage the men you know to overcome their uneasiness with prostate cancer screening and digital rectal exams in specific.

    o Explain to them how the potential benefits of screening, e.g. early detection, are worth the few seconds of an uncomfortable experience.

- If you have been affected by prostate cancer in anyway, directly or indirectly, speak out about your experience. Join support groups and help others with similar experience feel comfortable about opening up. Marianne Williamson wrote, "As we let our own light shine, we unconsciously give other people permission to do the same." It's time to let your light shine. Mr. Smith knows it, and so should you.

CHAPTER 11
I am a Survivor

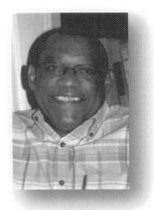

Lee Ashby, Retired

I'm originally from Indiana. I moved to Atlanta, Georgia in 1984. This was the best move I ever made. IBM brought me to Atlanta. My wife and I worked for IBM for a number of years. Basically, I'm a jack of all trades, master of none. I've also been a realtor for a number of years. The Atlanta area has been truly great for me.

I had prostate problems for years. I always went to a general practitioner who gave me a digital rectal exam, a prostate massage and a shot of penicillin. This cured the problems for a short time, but it always came back two, four or six months later and I'd go see the doctor again. Eventually, I heard about Dr. Bennett and he did basically the same thing when I initially saw him, but he also ran a series of tests. The PSA test came back high which led him to doing other things.

When I was 39 years old, I started to feel pain in my rectal area. I was having a pain running down my left leg all the way to my ankle. When I explained it to my general practitioner, he suspected prostate problems. After further examination, he told me I had an enlarged prostate. It would be many years before I came to see Dr. Bennett. The main reason I decided to see him was slightly disconcerting. When I went to urinate, it took me a good five minutes to even get it started. I knew something was wrong. My wife bugged me for years to go to an urologist. I put it off because I didn't think she knew what she was talking about. When I couldn't get my urine flowing, I stopped being stubborn. That's when we got the ball rolling.

Keep in mind, I only went to see a doctor when my prostate was bothering me. I didn't do annual physical exams. I don't know why. It wasn't about money because I've always had pretty good insurance. It was just something I put off and didn't do. It was something that should be done on an annual basis, and of course, I'm more diligent now. But it just was not something that I did then.

The very first day I saw Dr. Bennett, he did a PSA test and an ultrasound. The PSA was high, but the ultrasound didn't show anything. He scheduled me for a needle biopsy which came back positive. He called me in. My wife and I came in, and he broke the news to me: I had prostate cancer. At first, I thought I took it well. However, later on that night, I cried like a baby.

I've always been one to get a second opinion on anything that's as serious as what we were dealing with. I had Dr. Bennett release the slide to a friend of mine who is a physician in Indiana. He confirmed the diagnosis. At that point, I had to accept the grim truth. The phrase, 'you have cancer' is a dreaded phrase. It is something you never want to hear; and here it is, I'm facing it now. I have to deal with what the Lord gave me, and I have to deal with it in a positive manner and that's the bottom line. I've always been a positive type of individual, so I felt that Dr. Bennett and I could beat it. Not knowing how good Dr. Bennett was, I felt that I could beat it. That I along with my Jesus, could beat it. That's the way I took it. I cried, however, everything had to be positive after that.

I learned of my prostate condition on March 17, 1992. One month later, I had prostate cancer surgery. My wife was there, so of course, I tried to put that macho image up. She was my right hand even after surgery. She took care of me as well as anyone I know could have taken care of me. My daughter was still in elementary school, so she didn't really know what was going on with me. We were all very close; and my son – that's my man. I don't know what more to say, but he was there. He was there for sure.

Recently, some of my brother-in-laws have had some physical problems. They are in their 40's and 50's and they have never had a digital rectal exam. I think it's because they don't want anybody sticking anything in their rectum even though I've talked to them. I think it's a thing of homophobia. I've gone through it dozens of times, and I think it's uncomfortable. *Yes, the exam is uncomfortable.* But, after five to after five or 10 minutes, you're back to normal. Regardless of the fact that all of them know that I have had cancer – regardless that all of them know I have had 30 – 40 rectal exams, I cannot talk them into going to see a physician. It seems to me that it all comes down to that rectal exam.

The role of the spouse is very, very important. If it were not for the woman who is in your corner, pushing you to do certain things, nagging you to do certain things, a hard-headed male may never get it done. My wife pushed me to go to a urologist years before I actually did. Wives see things men just don't see. It's just that simple.

After prostate surgery, I missed having an ejaculation for about six months. You have orgasms, but you don't ejaculate anymore. That was a big emotional problem for me. I never told Dr. Bennett or anybody. In fact, all I told my wife was, I'm having problems.

Dr. Bennett told me about the support groups he was facilitating. He was helping groups of men who had prostate surgery. I went to one group and I listened to the guys. I was 43 years old, and I thought I was the youngest individual there. He told me there were individuals that were younger, but I hadn't met any. As I got more comfortable, the guys had me cracking up; they had me laughing. I realized that I wasn't the only one that was having problems. Finally, I realized that other individuals had problems which helped me a great deal. I never told anybody I had problems with ejaculation; I told people I had problems with prostate surgery. This was all psychological and eventually, that problem went away. I don't have a problem with it anymore.

I will soon be a 20-year survivor of prostate cancer. The thing I am most thankful for is that I got treatment. Without it, I may not be here today. I am glad to live to see my daughter who is taking the bar exam as we speak, struggle through law school -- and it has been a struggle. Without treatment, I may not have been here to see my daughter and my son graduate from college. I have not been blessed to have any grandchildren, but I know that's coming. It's great to see how well my offspring are doing. If it were not for Dr. Bennett and my wife pushing me to go to an urologist, I might not have seen any of this.

Discussion

Patients should be encouraged to be proactive about their prostate health. Failure to do so results in negative outcomes all too often. Mr. Ashby had chronic issues with his prostate; however, he continued to wait for symptoms before having his checkups. Although Mr. Ashby survived his ordeal, this is not the recommended route.

After being diagnosed with prostate cancer, Mr. Ashby elected to undergo a **radical prostatectomy** or total removal of the prostate gland. As with many forms of cancer, it is possible for the disease to appear down the line. This was the unfortunate case for Mr. Ashby. After his initial surgery, he needed to have external radiation therapy in order to eradicate traces of the disease in his body.

Facts

- In external radiation therapy, a large machine acts as the radiation source to target the general area where cancer is present. It differs significantly from brachytherapy (seeds) which involves the placement of radioactive prosthetics directly into the prostate gland.

- Radiation therapy is commonly given to radical prostatectomy patients 6-12 weeks postoperatively to minimize relapse.

    - In advanced cases, microscopic traces of prostate cancer can be found in the lymph nodes even after total removal of the prostate.

- As with most treatments of this disease, there are side effects that should be considered.

    - Acute side effects, or those that occur within the first 90 days of treatment, include: diarrhea, bloody stool, blood in urine, incontinence, and erectile dysfunction.

Recommendations

- Consult with a trusted physician to see if external radiation therapy is appropriate for you. Age and advancement of disease play a significant role in deciding treatment options.

- Choose a low-residue diet with foods that can be digested extremely easily. These can reduce frequent bowel movements or loose stool.

- If you have frequent diarrhea, replenish your hydration level by drinking significant amounts of fluids.

Medical Reference

Held-Warmkessel, Jeanne. Contemporary issues in Prostate Cancer: A Nursing Perspective (Jones and Bartlett Series in Oncology), 2000.

CHAPTER 12
Reality Check

Clifford Pauling

I was born and raised in New York City and moved to Atlanta 13 years ago. I came to Atlanta because of the slower pace, the style of living and New York money buys more here.

The first hint I had regarding prostate cancer was in 1996. I developed a urinary tract infection from holding my urine too long because I was unable to find a toilet. When I finally found one, urinating was painful. I assumed it was a temporary circumstance. When it continued, I reluctantly went to my primary care doctor. I had not gone to the doctor for years because I never got sick.

Since I was 62 years of age, the doctor asked if I had taken a PSA test recently. I did not know about PSA testing and that it was performed with a simple blood test. I had not had a medical checkup in over five years. My doctor conducted the PSA along with other laboratory tests. I was diagnosed with a urinary tract infection and my PSA result was 20 ng/mL.

I was never sick and I had no health issues at all. I was a runner and considered myself to be in excellent health. After the PSA, the doctor said, "You know, it's only supposed to be 4. I'm going to send you to a urologist." The doctor gave me some antibiotics and the PSA went down to 11. The doctor said it was still too high and ordered a biopsy.

Here's the funny story about the biopsy. I was going on vacation to the Grand Canyon in Arizona, so I asked if I could call to get my results. I called the doctor's office and said, "How's my test?" I was told, "Oh, everything is fine." I came home to find my answering machine full of 'Call us as soon as you can' messages. When I called, they asked me to come in. I thought they needed to take more tests. I went in and they said, "You have prostate cancer." I went into shock.

I thought I was going to die the next week or something. They said I needed to do some tests such as a bone scan and all this other stuff. I agreed to do everything because I was in a state of shock. However, the next day when I finally calmed down, I said, "I'm not doing anything, I don't want the tests." The people who were going to conduct the tests kept calling me. I figured they were calling because it was a very expensive test and they just wanted to make some money. They had scheduled me for surgery and a whole bunch of stuff, but I ended up not doing anything. After about a week or two, my sister said, "Why don't you consider going to Mexico and do one of those treatments there?" I passed on that as well.

For about six months, I didn't do anything but "watchful waiting." Then, I decided to get a second opinion from a urologist. The urologist waited until my PSA rose to 13 before deciding to do a biopsy. I did not tell him he was a second opinion. The urologist did a sonar directed biopsy, taking eight samples; he did not find any cancer cells.

The doctor said, "Your prostate is enlarged, but I'm not really concerned about the PSA. It's high, but let's watch and see what happens." I went back to him every six months for a year and a half and it stayed the same.

After moving to Atlanta, my PSA elevated to 26 or 29. I read that stress could cause that to happen. Rationalizing again, I attributed it to the stress of moving to Atlanta. I told myself, "You're in great shape, and you've got a PSA of 29." That's when I came to Dr. Bennett. He did a biopsy and found the cancer. Because the PSA was so high, he said he wanted to look at the lymph nodes. He found a microscopic presence in one of my lymph nodes. Dr. Bennett explained that the cancer had left the prostate and had gone to another part of the body. He wasn't sure where, but it was definitely in the lymph nodes. After he removed the lymph nodes, he said, "You don't have much choice with regard to treatments. You can't have surgery because it's metastasized, so we can't do it."

The only thing left to do was triple hormone therapy. Dr. Bennett explained that the triple hormone therapy was going to make me not like females. He said, "You're going to forget about women." I said, "Are you kidding? The horniest guy on this earth is going to forget about women?" I had to take pills twice a day and get a shot every three or six months. The pills were $220 a month, and I told Dr. Bennett, "Look, I want to live, but I have a choice: don't eat, live in the street, take this medication, or die." He said that I should contact the pharmaceutical company because they had a plan for people who can't afford it. Unfortunately, the pharmaceutical company said my income was too high.

I'm a disabled veteran, so I went to the VA Hospital and asked them to get me the medication. They agreed to give it to me for $4 a month. The shots were $1600 a shot. The insurance company paid for the shots, but wouldn't pay for the pills. I took the pills and the shots and Dr. Bennett's prediction was more than on-target. I didn't even notice women walking down the street and I'm a single guy who's been single for a long time. I didn't notice women and I didn't know that I didn't notice women. I just wasn't interested. I had a girlfriend and nothing was happening with her, so eventually we broke up.

The hormone treatment went on for about a year and it was the most devastating experience of my life. I was a world-class runner and in a master's program for people over 40. I was nationally and internationally known. After taking that treatment, I started having all kinds of physical problems. I have ten steps to take to get into my house. By the time I got to the tenth step, I was leaning on the railing. I used to run everything from 100 meters to the marathon. I had done eight marathons, a 26.2 mile race. Now, I couldn't walk up

10 steps to my house without breathing hard. I couldn't drive at night because I had vision problems. I was getting night sweats, hot flashes, developing breasts and couldn't sleep at night. Between the insomnia and feeling tired all the time, I didn't have any energy at all.

During a support group meeting at Dr. Bennett's office, a radiation oncologist came to speak to the group. Since Dr. Bennett said my cancer could be anywhere and radiation was not a treatment option, I asked the oncologist about my condition. He agreed to look at my file and discuss if there were any other options. We developed a bit of a friendship because we had a lot in common. I have three girls and the joke between us was: "Do you think God punishes guys like us by giving us girls?" At any rate, we tried a procedure where it was wide beam radiation. The oncologist radiated an area in my body larger than what's normally radiated so that he could cover the area of the lymph node. That worked and I got off the medication. A few weeks after I stopped taking the medication, I felt 100 percent better and eventually got back to my normal activities. My vision improved and my breasts disappeared. I didn't get back to my sexual activity because maybe I wore it out. That high level of activity never came back. So I had to find alternatives for that.

I never got back to my high level of competition in running. I did run some races after that but it was at a mediocre level. It's hard to fall from grace. That's a very hard thing. You step out there on the track and everybody's like, "Oh, there's Cliff;" and then Cliff comes in way in the back, you know? I had to acknowledge the fact that I'm not ever going to get back to that level of competition because all this stuff had taken a toll on my body.

My advice to men, especially Black men is that you should see your physician on a regular basis and try to be informed. I was 62 years old and I had never heard of a PSA. I find that inexcusable because I called myself well-read and knowledgeable. However, I didn't know anything about a PSA. You're supposed to check that after age 40, and here I was 62. I attribute that to the fact that I never went to a doctor. I hadn't had a checkup in about 10 years. I never caught a cold; I never had any reason to go to a doctor. I always felt that when you're sick, you go to a doctor. If you're not sick, leave it alone.

As a result of my experience, I have been extremely diligent in meeting my annual checkups to have a digital rectal exam, a prostate specific antigen test (PSA) and a complete physical exam. My most recent PSA was .34 ng/mL. I currently do not have any health issues and I am not on any medication. My blood pressure is currently 106/65 and my heart rate is 56 [bpm]. I recently had a hip replacement; therefore, I do not run anymore, but I exercise and ride my bike.

I have a lot to be thankful for. Like I said, I've had a charmed life. I've worked in several different fields which were all wonderful. I had what I call my fantasy job as a biomedical engineer. I've traveled around the world setting up clinics in developing countries. I've been to about 60 or more different countries and I have so many things to be thankful for. I have a wonderful family. I have a birthday this month and I'm going to be 77. Well yeah, that's my story and I'm sticking to it.

Discussion

Patients like Mr. Pauling, who have advanced prostate cancer (or cancer that has spread outside of the prostate) undergo androgen deprivation therapy, referred to as ADT, or more commonly known as hormone treatment. There are many variations of this type of treatment, but all involve using medication to suppress the hormonal mechanisms that help tumors to grow, i.e. male hormones (androgens). Otherwise, in more layman's terms, hormones are deprived of the necessary nourishment needed to survive. The most commonly known male androgen is testosterone. Many prostate cancer cells need testosterone to grow; therefore, inhibiting testosterone can impede the progress of an advancing cancer.

Drugs: Your doctor may suggest a drug that can block natural hormones.

- **Luteininizing hormone-releasing hormone (LH-RH) agonist:** These drugs prevent testicles from making testosterone.
- **Anti-androgens:** These drugs can block the action of male hormones.
- **Other drugs:** Some drugs can prevent the adrenal gland from making testosterone.

Androgen deprivation treatment can be accomplished in a variety of ways:

- It can be used as a first-line therapy in the form of an injection.
- It can be used as an injection along with an anti-androgen pill.
- Testicles can be surgically removed to achieve androgen deprivation (orchiectomy).
- Treatment can be used intermittently or continuously depending on the needs of the patient.
- It can be used after an initial treatment of surgery or radiation.

Along with most treatments, there are risks involved and they are likely to affect one's quality of life. After hormone therapy, side effects may include:

- Impotence
- Hot flashes
- Loss of sexual desire
- Weaker bones
- Breast growth
- Nausea
- Loss of appetite
- Diarrhea

Patients who experience a diagnosis of prostate cancer spreading outside of the prostate undergo treatment options as mentioned above. Due to the aggressiveness of Mr. Pauling's cancer, after a biopsy was performed and because his PSA level was so high, it was recommended that he undergo a lymph node dissection. During this procedure, lymph nodes near the prostate gland were removed and evaluated to determine if the prostate cancer has spread beyond the gland. After it was determined that Mr. Pauling's cancer had indeed moved outside of the prostate, he under went external or wide beam radiation therapy. The therapy was successful and kept Mr. Pauling's PSA level down and low.

After a few years of follow-up, if Mr. Pauling's PSA were to rise again, he could undergo intermittent hormone therapy. Intermittent therapy is used for a duration of six to twelve months where a low PSA level/value is maintained. The drug is then stopped until the PSA rises to a predetermined level. At this point, the drug is restarted. Often, this option is preferred for men who have advanced prostate cancer because it allows them to return to near normal levels of testosterone, potentially enabling sexual function and other important quality of life measures before the next potential cycle begins. Not all men who have experienced hormone therapy resume cycles.

Facts

- Yes, undergoing hormone treatment will change some of your lifestyle habits, but the most important thing is that you are alive. You can make decisions and you are maintaining a low PSA level.

- Any treatment that lowers hormone levels can weaken your bones. It is important to speak with your doctor about medicines or dietary supplements that can reduce your risk of bone fractures.

Recommendations

- If faced with a diagnosis of advanced prostate cancer, ask your doctor for all options.

- There are side effects to treatment, but there are ways that you can cope with these side effects with support.

- Join a local support group to discuss your fears and concerns. You are not in this alone. Refer to the resources described in the appendix.

Medical Reference

American Cancer Society. Cancer Reference Information: Hormone Therapy. 2005.

FACT:

"Many men don't find out they have prostate cancer until the cancer has spread, making it more difficult to treat."

CHAPTER 13
Becoming a Champion!

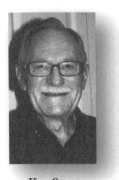

Ken Stevens
Georgia Prostate Cancer Coalition

I'm a college graduate with a B.A. in physics from the University of Denver combined with the University of Colorado. I played football at the University of Colorado. I got kicked out of school because I liked football, beer and women and ignored the academic requirement of school. They asked me to leave for a while, and I enlisted in the Marine Corps. I spent four years in the Marines and came out as a rocket scientist.

I came to Atlanta more than 45 years ago. I sold computers back when computers were not user-friendly. Now that they are user-friendly, I don't know anything about them. Twenty years ago, I got involved with the Cancer Society as a side gig.

I went in for an insurance examination and had a digital rectal exam. The best thing that ever happened to me was after Dr. Stubbs told me to go see a urologist because of a lump on my prostate; I did. That's when I had my first biopsy. A year later, I had another biopsy. This time I had the benefit of an ultrasound to guide the biopsy and the doctor found unequivocal cancer.

When I found out that I had prostate cancer, it didn't bother me a bit. I felt that it was something that you go do something about and get rid of it. My wife, a nurse at Shepherd Clinic, later said the reason I felt that way was because I didn't have a clue. She was very right. The second time I was told that I had prostate cancer, that it had returned and that the surgery had been unsuccessful, I had a breakdown. When my doctor, Sam Graham, told me that I had cancer again, he had tears in his eyes and I think that really impacted me. If he's afraid, I got to be afraid. That really, really, really sent me down. I went into a depression I'd never experienced before, and it was scary. I went to work and smiled, but nobody knew that I was about to kill myself.

I was on a panel at Emory University for the American Cancer Society. As we were fielding questions from the audience, for some reason, I started speaking about this fear that I had. I didn't know what I was afraid of at the moment. One minute, it's there, but nothing is wrong, and then all of a sudden an anvil gets dropped on me.

If you don't believe in angels, I can tell you they are there. My condition is that I have advanced microscopic metastatic, Stage 4 prostate cancer. I'm under treatment with hormone therapy right now and have been for about five years. To start with advanced prostate cancer, you have to go back to the beginning to figure out when that was.

The story of my diagnosis started out with a near-miss detection in 1987, so I've had cancer now for 24 years. The first time we found fibrous material because we didn't have ultrasound guided biopsy needles, and we didn't use PSA as a detection device. When I had my first biopsy, it was a three-day affair. The first day to find out how clean I was and to give me antibiotics to make sure I didn't have an infection. The next day was in a full-blown operating room with an anesthesiologist. It sounds kind of funny today because it takes 20 minutes to do it nowadays. They found fibrous material but it was not noted as prostate cancer.

A year later, I went back to the doctor and found a lump on my prostate with a digital rectal exam. According to the biopsy, it turned out that I had unequivocal prostate cancer. We started treatment at that time. A year later (1989), I had a radical prostatectomy. I actually reached Dr. Graham through Dr. James Bennett. My wife was a rehabilitation nurse at Shepherd Center, and she knew Dr. Bennett through his work in urology at the center.

About five years later, I found out that I was still maintaining my PSA test. The PSA has always been a diagnostic device, but we started using it because of the success rate as a detection device. Bad mistake. Now we know; back then it was the thing to do. We found out that my PSA was now increasing which meant I still had prostate cancer cells in my body. The doctor told me that I would have to have external radiation. This was to radiate the area around where the prostate used to be in order to keep it from spreading out since I didn't have any signs of it in my blood flow. I had no evidence as the CAT scans couldn't find it. I was classified at Stage 4, N0, T0. The scans couldn't find it, but there were cancer cells in my body somewhere. I had external radiation, a standard 37-day treatment at Emory University. That caused substantially more damage than surgery did. Since they had to radiate a rather large portion of supporting tissue and everything in the way using external accelerators to deliver the energy, the radiation burned everything and the cancer cells. It burned the neurons and nerve bundles; I have bone damage that was caused by the radiation, not the cancer. I started forming scar tissue; it took five to seven years before they started ratifying themselves into problems.

About 10 years after the radiation therapy, my PSA started going up. The velocity concerned us, so we started doing hormone therapy, ADT (Androgen Deprivation Therapy). I've been doing that ever since, as far as treatment is concerned. I really have not had any effect from the cancer in terms of my physiology. I can't point to a spot and say this is prostate cancer because I don't have a prostate or identifiable tumor anywhere in my body. However, we keep looking and maintaining because I want to know when it changes to the next phase. Because, there will be a next phase. Right now, my feet are on the green side of the grass. What more can I ask? I wake up in the morning, and my name is not in the obituary column. And man, I'm happy. There is no such thing as a 'bad day.'

Nobody was talking about prostate cancer when I got my prostatectomy, and I wondered why. I called the American Cancer Society and said, "Hey, look at the numbers. I've had this before, but I don't hear anyone talking about it. There's an awful lot of talk going on about breast cancer and they've got the same numbers – mortality, incidence, and so forth." I said, "How come we don't get any coverage?" They said, "Well, we don't talk about things like that." I've been talking about prostate cancer every since.

Here we are today, 23 years later. CNN did a live broadcast of my annual digital rectal exam. Dr. Graham pulled on his gloves (of course we were hidden by the table from the bottom parts), and faked performing a DRE. I said, "Dr. Graham, can you use another finger?" and he said, "Yeah, why?" I said, "I'd like a second opinion." And the cameraman about dropped his camera.

Ten years after I became a spokesman for the American Cancer Society, by talking about early detection, the message hasn't changed much. But, we've gotten away from that story into saying, some men get treated that shouldn't be treated. That's not the patient's fault, that's not the reason we shouldn't know whether or not something is going on in our body. Treatments are there. From experiences like mine, there are different things to do. They [the health professionals] modify it like a football game. You can modify your defense to meet the offense; everything is not going to be cool to start with.

I thought at the time, 10 - 11 years ago, that men needed to be more reasonable because all of the people that I met were going into an Alcoholics Anonymous Convention. This is where they sat around and talked about their problems. My attitude was, you don't really have problems. The guys who have problems are the ones that can't get to the convention and the ones that are dead. They've got problems and their families have problems. Prostate cancer is a family disease, so we have to work this out together.

The fact is, I've had prostate cancer and been in an advanced stage with it. I know what it does. I know that it can be treated from Stage 1 through Stage 4. I don't have cancer problems that I'm treating right now; I have problems with treatment from treatments: treating the side-effects of treatments with more treatments. So that's my physical problem.

It makes me upset that men don't know about prostate cancer – particularly men in the African-American community. The highest incidence of prostate cancer in the nation is in Georgia's South DeKalb County – it's the highest out there. Why should that be the case? It's hard to put an audience together to talk about prostate cancer. It's not the hottest item in the world to talk about. You learn that from your seminars. Men need to attend support groups and not be secretive about this. We need to talk about prostate cancer.

I've talked to men who say, "I might become impotent or incontinent." When I first heard this 10 or 15 years ago, I thought, *Lord, they're worried about incontinence.* There were ads on television. If they can have a great big Depends advertisement for women, we can do it. I mean, it's still a leak no matter how you put a bandage on it or a cork. You still have a problem.

When I first started talking about prostate cancer and early detection, Dr. Bennett said, "I want you to come down and go to an operation with me because if you're going to talk about this, you need to know about it." This was the best advice I ever had in my life. It was a great idea. I observed a cryotherapy procedure. The first thing I thought was, I used to work on Titan missiles. I am literally a rocket scientist.

I knew a lot about how missiles worked, how we transfer information and how we get cold stuff from one place to another. I was also amazed at how the console looked just like the one we used on rockets.

And I said, "Gee, this is fun." Dr. Bennett said, "See, I told you Ken would know what was going on here." It was very interesting how we put the liquid nitrogen into the prostate and freeze the prostate. I got to reach in and touch the prostate. From that type of experience, I learned the ramifications of treatment. You just think about it, that's cold stuff and it's not only freezing prostate cancer cells. It's not selective: it's freezing the whole doggone thing, so, there's gotta be a problem.

These are problems that can be overcome. The implant of radiation seeds is a great idea but this method has side effects. Surgery can present a problem, so everybody has a problem. There's no treatment that doesn't present a problem. Aspirin makes holes in your stomach. My job as I see it with the cancer coalition is to try to bring that state of awareness to a bunch of people that have a gland and don't know what it is, don't know where it is, don't know what it does and it doesn't hurt.

We've been brought up since children to rub some dirt on it and get back and play. It's okay; play it off or laugh it off. Unless the bone is sticking through the skin, we don't go to the doctor. We're men, macho and tough. You can't talk to a man and say, go to the doctor once a year. Why? I don't see any blood, there's nothing showing. The United States Preventative Task Force Services says, "Go to the doctor when you have symptoms." That's like saying, don't pay any attention to your smoke alarm, call the fire department when you see the flames in the attic. Well, that's just a little bit late. My responsibility is to make sure guys know what to do when they smell smoke.

Discussion: Advanced Prostate Cancer

If there needed to be an example for why men need to be screened regularly to monitor their prostate health, Mr. Stevens' story serves that purpose. Since the 1980's, he had been receiving regular screenings, and continued with a biopsy when his screening results were suspicious. The unfortunate irony is that his pro-activity was, nonetheless, rewarded with a diagnosis of prostate cancer.

The hallmark of advanced prostate cancer is **metastasis** or the spread of cancer cells to other parts of the body. Aggressive tumors escape the confines of the prostate gland, and frequently move to bones and lymph nodes. In these cases, the cancer is typically detected after a radical prostatectomy has been performed. After such a procedure, a patient's PSA value should be near zero, for they no longer have a prostate gland. Rising PSA values post-prostatectomy are a definite concern for the possibility of metastasis. Mr. Stevens continues to have microscopic, metastatic cancer which indicates that the locale of the spreading cancer cells is undefined.

Treatment options for metastatic prostate cancer differ drastically from those for cancer localized in the gland. Cryoablation and brachytherapy are not viable options because neither has an effect on the cancer cells outside of the prostate gland. Radical prostatectomy isn't typically recommended for viable patients because of the risk of releasing cancer cells into the rest of the body due to incomplete removal of the gland. Oncologists may recommend administering external radiation or hormonal therapy to destroy the cancerous cells that may be present in bones, lymph nodes, or other areas. Mr. Stevens was subject to both of these treatments in an attempt to control the growth of cells that could not be traced.

Most disconcerting about Mr. Stevens' journey is that, despite his conscientious efforts to prevent the development of cancer, he was still subject to the recurring disease. However, with every passing moment, knowledge regarding prostate cancer detection and treatment continues to increase. Mr. Stevens' story is a testament to the importance and urgency to get screened for the disease despite your fear.

Discussion: Becoming a Champion

Ken Stevens is a champion.

He won't receive a diamond-studded ring, nor go to Disney World. But, he is a champion. It is so easy to just fade into black when dealing with prostate cancer. It is easy to evade the elephant in the room with complacency. It is easy to accept fate's ill will, fold a bad hand and slide quietly out of the game. Something about Mr. Stevens, though, drives him towards the path unbeaten. If poker is the metaphor, Mr. Stevens took his only hand and went all in.

There is one very fundamental reason behind the silence of those affected by prostate cancer. The uncomfortable nature of the subject is a factor. Fear also plays a part. Our most extensive obstacle we face, is this contagion known as *silence*. The men chronicled in this book are pioneers in a relatively uncharted territory. **They are taking a leap of faith by offering their stories when** acceptance is such an uncertainty.

> *"Your playing small does not serve the world. There is nothing enlightened about shrinking so that other people won't feel insecure around you. We are all meant to shine as children do. We were born to make manifest the glory of God that is within us. It's not just in some of us; it's in everyone. And as we let our own light shine, we unconsciously give other people permission to do the same. As we are liberated from our own fear, our presence automatically liberates others."*

Marianne Williamson's famous quote could not be applied to a better scenario. It is the liberation of fear that is the key to true prostate cancer awareness. Speaking out, to be cliché, has a snowball effect. In the new age of communication that has incorporated social media, social causes gather support at rates unprecedented. National revolutions, economic theories and hilarious viral videos are all bolstered by the phenomenon of human communication in the 21st Century. Why is it, then, that we have failed to capitalize on the ease of knowledge distribution?

We have turned a blind eye towards the efforts of those carrying the torches for this cause. Unfortunately, blindness is a permanent condition. We can, however, use our functional eye to see what is happening with prostate cancer through the scope of the world to which our mind is already receptive. It is not human nature to place the interest of the majority after that of the remainder. The irony is that men, their wives and their families (i.e. those affected by prostate cancer) are *not* a minority in the simplest sense of the word! So why is it that a concern of this massive subcategory of society is not a concern of society as a whole? The answer is simple. *Society does not know.* To those who have witnessed the unchecked power of prostate cancer, we must take the responsibility to follow Mr. Stevens' lead, and educate ourselves and others on the topic. Once the fight for prostate cancer awareness is more public, the world will realize the effects of this disease are more far-reaching than anyone ever thought. The perception will be that men deserve to have attention brought to this issue. And in today's society, perception is reality.

A survivor is someone who managed not to lose. A champion is a winner. It is essential to make this distinction when determining how to pursue life with and after prostate cancer. There comes a crossroad where a man must decide if he will find a way not to die or if he will take ownership of and pride in his health in order to *live*. When the history books are written, will your story be one of a survivor or one of a champion? It is your duty to the world, your family and yourself to choose the latter.

Facts

- **Gleason Grade** 4 and 5 cancerous cells are considered advanced. (Different from **Gleason Score)**
- **Metastasis** to bones, bladder and other surrounding tissues is common in advanced prostate cancers.
- **External beam radiation** and **hormonal therapy** are treatments generally used for advanced prostate cancer.

Recommendations

- Continue to have prostate health exams annually including a PSA test and a DRE.

- Do not wait until you have symptoms to get checked. Monitoring a change in PSA proactively can lead to significantly earlier diagnoses, and an opportunity to prevent the advancement of the cancer.

Medical Reference

Oesterling, M.D., Joseph E. and Mark A. Moyad, M.P.H. *ABC's of Prostate Cancer.* Bayer Corporation, 1996.

FACT:

"In less than 100 minutes, another African American man will die from disease."

CHAPTER 14
Competing for Your Life

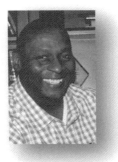

Curtis Lovejoy
Paralympic Medalist

I wasn't born disabled. I was injured in a car accident in 1986 on Veterans Day. As I was headed out on the expressway about 8:00 on a rainy morning, a car emerged onto Delowe Drive and came directly in front of me. I hit the brakes. The car hydroplaned, slammed into the guard rail and flipped over. I proceeded down the expressway like I was actually driving the vehicle. When I woke up, I ran directly into a pole. I broke the bone in my neck, fractured my left wrist, and was paralyzed from the neck down. I couldn't feel a thing but something like a blow torch in my lower back. A driver that was behind me told me the paramedics were on the way. When the Grady arrived, I remember one guy saying something like, "Man, he looks pretty bad; look at his feet; look at his wrist." I tried to move but I couldn't. They got me out, strapped me to the board and took me to Grady Hospital.

When we got to Grady, I couldn't turn my head that much, but I could turn my eyes and look sideways. I saw a lot of people in the hospital emergency room. I was wondering why they were looking after me and not looking after them. I heard one of the doctors whisper, "We can't do anything for him 'cause he has a spinal cord injury." That wasn't good news to hear at that time, but by the grace of God, I arrived at Shepherd Center the same day I got hurt. Normally, you don't get insurance the same day; it usually takes several weeks or months. I later learned after doing some research that Grady Hospital staff didn't know anything about treating people with spinal cord injuries. They didn't know about turning people every four hours or every six hours. A lot of people who went to Grady developed bed sores because they never turned them. The same day, 24 pastors came together very quickly and said we got to get him into Shepherd Spinal Center. I was admitted that evening.

I didn't know what was going on. When I thought about trying to move, I couldn't. The doctor took a piece of my pelvis, infused it in the neck and got me into a wheelchair. The doctor said, "Curtis, you'll never walk again." When he said that statement, I don't think I said another word for about three days. I would never be able to grab my wife by the hand and walk her down the street. A lot of thoughts ran through my mind. I tried to figure out where I went wrong. I was the district manager for a major fast food franchise and had 34 stores. I had about three or four thousand employees. I was a young guy who was a cocky, arrogant S.O.B. If you didn't do it my way, you didn't work for me.

Dr. Bennett was my first urologist at Shepherd Spinal Center. Here I am, a quadriplegic. I had a lack of sensation, but now my sensation has returned. My movement returned and the doctors didn't understand how I was able to walk when I didn't have a back muscle.

Dr. Bennett had this mission that he was on. He wasn't a very vocal man, and I used to wonder why this man didn't talk. As I got to know him better and the more that he learned about me competing and breaking a world record, he opened up his world to me.

I started coming in getting checked out by Dr. Bennett. Every time, he would say, "Everything is fine." This process kept going on and on. He used to call me Mr. Lover, the Love Man. A year ago, after getting my checkups, he did his normal testing and determined the PSA went down.

Prior to all of that, I noticed my burst of energy wasn't there in my competition. I noticed in 2008 when I went to China, my energy just wasn't there. The burst of energy just wasn't there. I kept saying, "what's wrong?" When I went to my physician at Shepherd Center, he started running all these tests. He said, "Everything's fine, Curtis. Maybe it's just you," I said, "No it ain't there, I know my body, it ain't there. Something is missing." After Dr. Bennett did all these tests, he called me and said, "I found a little spot, probably less than the size of an M&M." He said, "I think it's the prostate, but we're gonna do a bone scan and MRI." I said, "What's wrong, doc?" He said, "I don't know, we want to check you out to make sure you're okay."

All of those tests came back negative, and then finally he said we need to do surgery. Dr. Bennett gave me three options: radical prostatectomy, radiation therapy and cryosurgery. He said, "Can you still pee?" I said, "Yeah!" He said, "I can't give you the first three; I can give you the freeze." I said, "What are you talking about?" So he said, "I want you to think about which thing you want to do." After giving me the 411, now I am not in shock – I am surprised, but I'm not shocked. Because, I've always known that there's a war going on inside of our body.

We may never know when it's gonna take place or when it's going to surface. Dr. Bennett said, "You think about it and let me know." I left his office, sat in my van, had a little prayer, went back into his office and said, "I know what I wanna do. Let's go over the last one." He said, "You're sure?" I said, "Yeah." He said, "Did you talk to your wife?" I called her and I told her that I am going to have the surgery. She said, "Are you sure?" Dr. Bennett said, "When do you want to do it?"

Since I had to compete at the Georgia Dome on the 4th of July, I chose to have the procedure two days after the competition. My wife was content because she knew where her faith was and she knew where my faith was. My immediate family, sisters and brothers, couldn't handle it. They were on pins and needles, but here I was content. Then all of a sudden, my wife said, "I don't want you to have this nonchalant attitude like it's not a serious surgery." I said, "It might be a serious surgery but what can scare me more than my accident?" I faced death in my accident, so this ain't gonna scare me. I said, "When I was paralyzed from the neck down and didn't know if I was going to walk again, that was death. This is totally different. It's in God's hands."

I competed and won a gold medal. The following month, I was scheduled to go to the World Championship for swimming. Dr. Bennett was aware of my schedule. I went in on a Saturday, was prepped, followed by consultation with my Pastor. He told me, "Everything's going to be alright; you know what you have do." I said, "Yes sir." I began to tell Dr. Bennett, "Hey, I didn't sleep well last night 'cause I had to stop drinking liquid after 12:00 a.m." When I don't drink water, my legs go into spasms. My leg get jumpy when I don't have water. He said, "Let me tell you something, you leave the surgery to me and you do what you gotta do, alright?" The next thing I know, I was out.

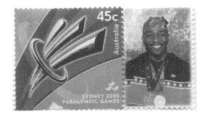

Curtis Lovejoy, turned tragedy into triumph. Despite a disheartening prognosis, Curtis went on to become a medalist in the Paralympic games, winning over 400 medals including nine Olympic medals, six of which are gold.

Regarding the number of medals I have won in swimming and fencing, I stopped counting and that was five years ago. I stopped because they don't faze me anymore. Because, my life has purpose now – changing people's lives. The first medal that I won, my father was standing right there with me. It was probably one of the most rewarding things because I am the last born of a family of 13 of parents who worked on a farm. My mother made it to the 8th grade. My father quit school in the 7th grade because he had to work on the farm. My parents wanted a better life for their children.

I still compete around the world and my prostate cancer is gone. I urge all Black men to get tested early and often. Early diagnosis and treatment can make the difference in life.

Discussion

Cryotherapy is a minimally invasive treatment option for men with localized prostate cancer. The procedure utilizes the guidance of special probes to subject the gland to extreme cold with the aid of liquid nitrogen to destroy abnormal tissues. Recent technology improvements have enabled the cryosurgeon to visualize the prostate gland while inserting the cryosurgical probes that utilize liquid nitrogen to distribute extreme cold to the intended tissues. See image of cryosurgery procedure in Figure 1.1.

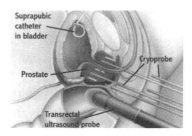

Figure 1.1: Image of cryosurgery procedure

This treatment is done under either general or local anesthesia and generally takes about two hours. The time allotted for this procedure is dedicated to the placement of probes in the prostate gland and the remainder for the freezing procedure and removal of the probes. To assist the surgeon in visualizing the gland, an ultrasound probe is placed in the patient's rectum. The surgeon then places approximately five cryoprobes through the perineum (the area between the bottom of the scrotum and the anus) into the prostate. Your prior treatment history will determine the amount of probes that will be required to treat the prostate.

Super-cooled liquid nitrogen is then circulated through the cryoprobes' tip and the prostate tissue is frozen. There are four different types of cryoprobes, each producing a different shaped ice ball. Each probe can be controlled independently. This allows the urologist to "sculpt" the ice ball or freeze zone very precisely. All the prostate tissue is frozen. The entire procedure is monitored in real time using ultrasound visualization. The urologist, therefore, can make sure all the prostate tissue is frozen but the non-prostate tissue such as the urethra and rectum is spared.

Simultaneously, the urethra's special tube, also a urethral warming catheter, circulates warm water and it is inserted into the urethra and passed into the bladder. Its job is to transfer heat into the urethra during the procedure, protecting the urethral tissue from the freezing temperatures used to treat the prostate.

Patients are able to leave the hospital within one to two days or possibly the same day if the procedure is performed in an outpatient facility. General follow-ups will occur for the next few months and years to monitor your prostate gland. The most common complication after surgery is sloughing, the shedding of dead tissue. This complication can cause urinary tract obstruction (blockage). Catheterization is a common method used to treat mild to moderate instances. Other complications include incontinence, fistulas and impotence. Cryotherapy is an attractive option to many patients who identify it as less invasive and risky than a radical prostatectomy.

Facts

Benefits to Consider

- Minimally invasive
- Choice of general or regional anesthesia
- Speedy recovery
- Great option for treatment if previous treatments have failed
- Can be repeated

Potential Complications to Consider (in descending rate of occurrence)

- Impotence (partial or total loss of erection) due to freezing
- Incontinence (partial or total loss of urinary control)
- Fistula (abnormal opening between two organs)

Recommendations

- Educate yourself on treatment options
- Seek out support from family and friends

FACT:

"The key to the successful treatment of any cancer is early diagnosis."

CHAPTER 15
The Fear Factor

Anthony Holland

I am a native of Atlanta, born in 1958 – a Grady Baby – the youngest of four. I initially came to see Dr. Bennett because of frequent urination and pressure in my lower stomach region. I had never had a urological exam prior to that. No, [we] stay away from that. However, I did have regular exams.

My first thoughts when I was given the diagnosis were interesting because I talk about this a lot. I walked out of [Midtown Urology] like I was wading through Jell-O. It was a total shock! They had done an earlier biopsy, and it came back negative. That had been a couple of years before my diagnosis. When I came in, they told me that my PSA was elevated, and they wanted to do another biopsy. I said to myself, okay, no big deal, we've done this before. I really wasn't thinking about it, and then, there was that little bit of thought that maybe they will find something. It was two weeks before my return visit to find out the results. I felt if they had found something, they would have called and said come on in earlier. I really walked in there not expecting anything.

You know, it's funny; I can't really say that there was a fear. My general fear was that I was just past my 40's and it seemed like everything was falling apart. As far as any fears about reproductive health or anything like that, that wasn't even on the radar. I wasn't even thinking about that.

The day I learned I had prostate cancer was a comedy of errors. I will never forget that day. I got my diagnosis on June 6, 2006. I was 48. I came in to see the doctor at about 9 o'clock in the morning. After I left there, I was to go to my aunt's funeral. I spent the rest of that day saying to myself, okay, this is not your story, this is not your story, and this is not your story. So that kind of added to it all. I don't know that there was immediate fear – there was more shock than fear. I had always been a bookworm, so I knew from my reading that this [prostate cancer] was treatable. Depending on what stage you're in, this is treatable. That helped stop the fear, too, and [it] immediately sent me to where I've always found comfort, to books and to the Internet.

My maternal grandfather died of colon cancer. When some of the fog cleared, I thought about it. I thought, okay, I bet this is where that started. Of course, he died back in the early sixties; it was a very big possibility that when it had been in the prostate, it had been missed, and by the time it showed up, it was colon cancer. That was somewhat confirmed for me when two years later, in 2008, my brother was diagnosed. He is doing okay with the physical part of it, but, with the psychological part, he's not doing so well.

I thought about my brother a lot. He, like the rest of us, went to the doctor only when something was wrong. The fact that I had my diagnosis first and talked to him, I think it alarmed him somewhat, when he got his diagnosis. It didn't frighten him as bad as it would have. I remember when I first told him about my diagnosis, he looked at me and said, "Oh great, you can't live without your prostate, can you?" I understood that fear because we are the last surviving from our nuclear family; it's just him and me. There was that thought in the back of our mind that something's going to happen to one of us and whoever's left will be all alone. I understood that fear but I think my experience has helped him around that part of it.

My message to Black men today would be that general care and routine checkups have to become a way of life. It's not something that we can continue to run from. We hear about women having to have pap smears and mammograms; this is just as important for us as those things are for women. This is a part of our lives, whether we like it or not. And it's a school of thought that all men will get this sometime, it's just a matter of when. It's got to become that open and revealed to people. As far as the longstanding joke about the finger in the anus, if it comes down to saving my life, then I got to do what I got to do.

I would like to see more information directed towards post-operative effects for all men. But even more than that, I feel like there needs to be some attention given to the younger man who has not had children; address those things for him. What happens to the man who is single, who's not in a relationship? Dating is not what it was before the loss of my prostate. All spontaneity in sexual encounters is gone, and people need to know that. You need to know that you have to plan for sex. It can't just be spur-of-the-moment. People have to get their heads around that. When I get back into a relationship, because that will be the first relationship I've been in since my prostate surgery, how will I handle that?

One of the things that I will say, my brother and I have had a chance to talk about dating relationships with prostate issues. There's a whole different type of pressure for him because he had just started a relationship when this happened, and now there's a lot of different emotions going on there. It makes him feel inadequate sometimes; he feels like he can't please his partner and that she may start to look elsewhere. All these are things that, whether we like it or not, are tied to this issue so there needs to be some support out there.

I don't know that anything can be done to rectify our lack of knowledge other than education, talking to people and helping them to understand that this is a part of life. This is an area, to me, where we have to get out of our own way. We have to recognize that this is what it is; we are not invincible. We need to pay attention to the fact that this can and will likely happen to us at some point in time. So, what do we do? What's our game plan? The other thing that I think is very important is that along with talking about what may happen or what could happen, we also have to arm people and tell them what to expect when it does happen.

Yes, there were side effects; I couldn't get hard. How do I turn this into a learning experience? [How do I] pay attention to what's going on with me, with my body, and what happened after this? I learned a lot about this, that I never expected to learn. I learned a lot about what happens afterward, the fear that came. I didn't know what to expect because I'd never been here before. That's why I feel that support groups are so important. I don't think anybody can give you information as well as somebody that's been there.

Discussion

Erectile dysfunction (ED) is defined as the persistent inability to achieve and/or maintain an erection sufficient for satisfactory sexual activity and is a common problem in the male population over the age of 40. ED, to some degree is estimated to affect up to 30 million men in the United States. Despite the fact that ED is extremely common, less than 2 in 10 (20%) are seeking treatment because of fear. It is often difficult for a man to discuss erectile dysfunction, or the possibility thereof, with their sexual partner and health provider.

Incidence increases with age: about 5 percent of 40-year-old men and between 15 and 25 percent of 65-year-old men experience ED, but it is not an inevitable part of aging.

Nevertheless, it is very important that if you have ED that you seek treatment and get treated because it is treatable. It may even uncover other serious, treatable disorders. It is important for you to speak up about your concerns to your physician. Don't ever assume that ED is a natural consequence of aging. You may be doing yourself a disservice.

Treatments for Erectile Dysfunction

Oral medications: As noted below, there are a number of medications available that may improve blood flow to the penis. When combined with sexual stimulation, this can produce an erection.

- Viagra ™ (sildenfil citrate)
- Cialis™
- Levitra™
- Staxyn™

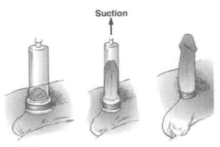

Osbon ErecAId ®

Vacuum Pump Therapy: As illustrated above, an erection can be gained using a vacuum system. To ensure the therapy works, a tube is placed over the penis. Then the pump creates a vacuum to draw blood into the penis, causing an erection. A tension band is placed around the base of the penis to hold in the blood.

Intraurethral suppositories: A suppository that contains medication is inserted into the urethra.

- MUSE

Injection Therapy: Drugs utilized with injection relax the blood vessels and let blood flow into the penis. Within 10 to 15 minutes, the penis can become rigid enough for sexual intercourse.

- Trimix
- Edex

Penile Implant: When medications are exhausted, then surgical approaches are entertained. During surgery, an implant is placed inside the spongy chambers of the penis. Examples include:

- *Semi-rigid or malleable rod implants:* Easy to use and bendable rods can make the penis appear erect. When not in use, the rods can be bent downward. See diagram on next page.

- *Fully inflatable implants:* The implant is easy to use in one fast and simple one-step deflation. It is totally concealed in the body. It requires manual dexterity and training to enable one to use the pump properly.

- *Three-piece prosthesis:* Acts and feels more like a natural erection. It also can expand the girth of the penis and appear more firm and full than the other implants. It feels softer and more flaccid when deflated. It does require manual dexterity and possibility of unintentional erections.

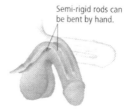 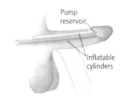 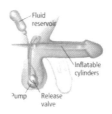

Many physicians still maintain that if ED were important to patients, then they would bring up the issue of ED during their medical visits; however, data has shown clearly that patients are waiting for the doctor to initiate a discussion on ED.

Erectile Dysfunction screenings **may** signal underlying disease such as:
- Diabetes
- Hypertension
- Dyslipidemia
- Certain malignancies

Erectile Dysfunction can be associated with:
- Morbidity
- Anxiety and depression
- Decreased self-esteem
- Negative effect on relationships

Maintaining and possessing a healthy sex life should be a standard for both men and women; however, men who suffer from Erectile Dysfunction usually feel discouraged and depressed. Now is the time to be your own advocate and speak to someone about your concerns.

Support groups provide an atmosphere of understanding. Each person in the group has either been through the fire or is concerned with the road ahead. Because of this mutual comprehension factor, members are able to be completely express themselves regarding their insecurities. As Mr. Holland so insightfully noted, women are open with the maintenance of their health. It has been a ritual for them since they were very young, and it is necessary for men to do the same.

As men, we typically like to surround ourselves with responsibilities and tasks in order for us to appear less vulnerable to emotional disturbances. Our psyches are so guarded that when something breaks through the barrier, we don't know how to react. Typically, we can always rely upon the support of our family, our spouses and our friends. The viability of that support system, however, is contingent upon our willingness to communicate our distress.

Prostate cancer is a silent killer. Not because it takes lives without offering warnings, but because it demoralizes its victim to the point where he encloses himself in a shell of doubt, away from family, away from friends. Mr. Holland was a single man with very little immediate family when he was diagnosed with prostate cancer. Self-education consoled his uneasiness about the physical symptoms of the disease, not the psychological.

After his diagnosis, Mr. Holland realized that the only way he would be able to come to terms with both the physical and psychological shortcomings of his condition would be to express his sentiments to other people. Unlike the stereotypical man, Mr. Holland was no stranger to therapy sessions, so he sought help from support groups hosted by his diagnosing urologist office. There he could share his story with other affected men who were also struggling with acceptance.

Facts

- Erectile Dysfunction affects 1 in 5 men and over 30 million American men.
- 70% of ED patients fail to bring up the issue and a number of physicians don't ask the question.
- Support groups are not for the effeminate male or for men who are more in tune with their emotions as stereotypes suggests. It is for the male who wants answers and wants support to get through a tough time in his life.

Recommendations

- If you are unable to maintain an erection, **speak up,** and let your physician know. There is no reason you should keep your silence.
- Join a support group. Hear and gain the advice of men who are dealing with the effects of prostate cancer just like you.

Medical Reference

Oesterling, M.D., Joseph E. and Mark A. Moyad, M.P.H. *ABC's of Prostate Cancer.* Bayer Corporation, 1996.

CHAPTER 16
I am not a Survivor!

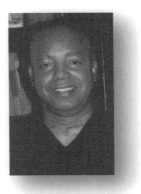

Cassius Williams, Retired

I graduated from high school in 1958, attended an HBCU and completed a master's degree in Mathematics. I married my wife Connie, a beautiful, special, talented and virtuous angel 49 years ago. We are proud parents of a son and daughter. We also have one grandson.

After having taught mathematics and science in the public school system for three years, I worked for an insurance company for 30 years. I coached basketball during my teaching years, played basketball in high school and at 71 years old—I'm still playing today. I am looking forward to continuing as long as I am able.

Working for an insurance company allowed me to be more aware of the need for annual physicals and checkups, including a regular annual review of my PSA scores. I monitored what I considered an acceptable score range, below 2, during my 30's and 40's. The score stayed around 4 or less in my 50's. My score began to rise a little in my late 50's, but never greater than 4.7; and thus I was never overly concerned.

In June 1999, I went in for a routine checkup with my urologist, Dr. James K. Bennett. After testing and reviewing my history, he recommended a biopsy. That was when the evidence of prostate cancer was found.

Needless to say, I was guilty and overwhelmed by the finding. I was in denial and did not believe it. I thought I was doing a good job of testing regularly and keeping up with my score. I certainly thought a score of 4.7 was safe. I just could not believe the biopsy was accurate. After receiving second opinions from several doctors and results, I was convinced the evidence was real.

When I continued to meet with Dr. Bennett, I finally said to him, "I wanted to see the evidence of what he saw that convinced him that I had prostate cancer." He said, "I've never been asked that before." I said, "I'm sorry, but I'm still dealing with denial, I guess." And he said, "What do you mean by that?" I said, 'Whatever you saw that convinced you that I have it, I would like to see it too." And he said, "Okay, I guess you would have to see the slides then."

We went to the hospital laboratory to view the slides in the microscopic instrument that showed me the results of the biopsy. I could see that my left side prostate was more impaired and looked nothing like my right side. I was sure that there was something different. And then, my wife, daughter and I, continued to have interviews with Dr. Bennett and decided that we would proceed. At that point, six months had passed; I had wasted six months of my life by procrastinating.

Treatment didn't trouble me anymore since I was hyped after six months of procrastinating with little or no sleep. I was just depressed and distressed and just in disbelief about it. However, the evidence was enough for me to take action, and so we decided to proceed. I had been versed on all of the options, and I had read about them. I had seen five other doctors, and their opinions were consistent as well. We agreed that I would take the least evasive procedure, which [I felt] was the seed implantation. I barely recall the procedure. It was painless.

My nature is to be inquisitive, and I'm generally that way with most things. I guess it's just my analytical background; I'm a math major and I just want to know more about what makes it right, what makes it real. Dr. Bennett once said, "You ask more questions than most patients I ever see,"

When my surgery was over, I asked how everything went. He said, "I knew you were going to ask that. I'll tell you how everything went after you can go to the men's room and pee. Because if you can pee, I'm gonna let you go home." All I could think was, *please let me pee.* I went to the bathroom and there it was. I was able to urinate and an hour and a half later, I was back at my house.

I have accepted myself now as an ambassador for the cause. I feel like I should share with others my experience. First and foremost, [you must] be active in terms of being tested and be aware of the likelihood that every man will have it if he lives long enough, and that he doesn't have to be any particular age. But if they test regularly, then that's really number one, in spite of all the controversies now about it. I believe that the test is a vehicle that can help men, along with the doctors, to determine to some extent what's going on down there.

Number two, I would say to be obedient to the medical advisors in terms of what they prescribe you to do, in terms of caring for it, maintaining and providing good maintenance for not only the prostate but for all of the organs of the body. And number three, if you are in fact diagnosed with prostate cancer, please accept it as reality. You should accept it as real and take whatever steps to eradicate it or to get it taken care of, and to believe that it can be; and that it's not a death sentence.

I was 58 when I was diagnosed with prostate cancer. I'm now 71. The sun has been shining a little brighter these last 13 years. The regrets I have are that I was such a procrastinator about the evidence, and not having believed what I was told and accepting it as just a bump in the road. I regret that I did not just proceed to get treatment, knowing if it was the Lord's will, I would be healed and that life would go on as it should be the rest of the days of my life.

Discussion

While Mr. Williams was telling his story, he brought up a very interesting point. He said, "I am not a prostate cancer survivor. Don't call me that! The word *survivor* implies that this is something that I was supposed to die from." He was right. Survivors seem to manage their way out of hopeless situations, drawing from the power of their own resolve. Although the nature of prostate cancer may imply a dire situation, life with, or after, prostate cancer does not have to be fruitless.

It is very common for a person, man or woman, to be overcome with this feeling of hopelessness. Hopelessness can manifest itself in our daily lives in a plethora of ways; however, the tendency to mentally, physically, and socially shut down is even more prevalent. Each of these aspects of human life is important in its own respective manner. It seems, though, that maintaining oneself physically can impact the other factions of life. Physical activity is, as defined by the National Cancer Institute, a component of the energy balance, along with weight maintenance and diet.

To be sure, Mr. Williams is a specimen. There are very few men of age 70 that maintain a level of activity comparable to his. It is evident that his passion and competitive nature have a significant effect on his morale and his zeal even into his retirement years. Most impressive about his continued physical activity is that he managed to enthusiastically exercise *after* his incidence with prostate cancer. It is known that this kind of rigorous exercise is critical to a person's overall health. But, what effects does it have on the progression of the disease experienced by a prostate cancer patient?

Although there has been no biological determination of a mechanism of action, there is an association of diet and exercise with the behavior of cancer within the body that cannot be ignored.

As mentioned earlier, diet selection serves a similar role in health maintenance with and without cancer. The etiology or cause of prostate cancer cannot conclusively be connected to a man's diet; however, it is important to his overall health which manifests itself as quality of life with or without a prostate cancer diagnosis.

Facts

- For men age 65 and older, studies have shown that those who participate in regular vigorous activity are at a lower risk of aggressive prostate cancer. They are also at a lower risk of dying from prostate cancer.

- There are claims that diets with high fat content lead to a higher risk of aggressive prostate cancer although contemporary research has proven inconclusive on this issue.

- Adding flavones to your diet can decrease your risk of developing the disease. Flavones are found in many cereals and herbs and contribute, not only to reduction of prostate cancer risk, but overall health as well. Soy is another source of flavones that is readily available.

Recommendations

- Make any attempts to remain active throughout your life. Whether you're taking a walk, playing basketball or just stretching while you watch television; physical activity is essential to maintaining your health.

- Create a diet that is healthy in nature and low in saturated fat. Whether or not you will prevent your prostate cancer doing this is highly debatable, but you *will* be a healthier person regardless of the status of your prostate. Try to include soy if possible!

- Although PSA level of 4 ng/mL or below is considered normal, a man who presents with a statistically normal PSA level can still have prostate cancer. Refer to Chapter 4 for more information regarding PSA screening.

Medical References

Giovannucci, M.D., Sc.D., Edward L., Yan Liu, MS; Michael F. Leitzmann, M.D., Meir J. Stampfer, M.D., Dr.P.H., Walter C. Willett, M.D., Dr.P.H. A Prospective Study of Physical Activity and Incident and Fatal Prostate Cancer. *Archives of Internal Medicine*. 2005; 165: 1005-1010. May 9, 2005.

Chapter 17
The Check Up

Bishop Thomas Alvin Body

I was born in Dallas, Texas and raised in the briar patch. I came to Atlanta in 1983 from Minnesota traveling as an evangelist. I enjoy living in Atlanta as a pastor and psychologist at One Accord Church in Decatur, Georgia: W*here a stranger meets a friend and a sinner meets God.*

For me, the battle with prostate cancer was sort of insignificant because I was having a checkup every year and my PSA was checked during those times. This time it was elevated a little and Dr. Bennett had been very cautious. He said, "come on in, let me do a biopsy and see what is going on." Sure enough, there was a bit of cancer there. It was not as frightening because I had read so much, and I knew so much about how prostate cancer can be cured if it's discovered early enough. God was guiding me.

My family became very protective of me. My wife is not the kind of person who can be a straightforward nurse. She would be a nurse that would let you feel good if you were dying, and she would never ever let you know how she really felt about it. She was very helpful. We just said, "Let's do it" and I went on to have the surgery. I'm 78 years old, and I enjoy everything. I can't run like I used to run – I can't do all the things I did as a young man. But I can do all the things an old man can do and enjoy my wife.

I am thankful to the Lord primarily because he has guarded me all my life and things just don't sneak up on me. I've had some surprises, but with things like this, there has been a forewarning. That is why I started having checkups every year. I asked Dr. Gander who's a cardiologist, "Am I a hypochondriac?" He said, "No, you're just the type of person who watches your body and it's good to watch your body and what type of things you put into your body."

Many men are uncomfortable about the digital rectal exam. It's easier to accept when you understand that the payoff of the examination exceeds the discomfort of the examination. It's a lot better than having cancer. It's much more easily received if you pay attention to the outcome and not the examination.

There has been a lot of concern about Black men not having annual checkups. Somehow or another, I feel this goes back to slavery. As Black men, we had been in slavery for hundreds of years in the strictest sense of slavery. Black men are still under a slave mentality. A slave doesn't say very much; he only performs He works every day, gets the food and all that goes into making a living for his family. He doesn't have much to say and doesn't get very much on Father's Day and Christmas; he gets a pair of socks and a handkerchief. But I think the quietness is due to a cultural kind of thing that keeps us denying the reality of what's going on with us. We don't want to really find out that we have cancer. I would rather not know that I have cancer than to know that I have cancer and try to do something about it. I guess it's sort of a wish list; that I can avoid having cancer by my ignorance of it.

The woman expects so much from the man; he's the breadwinner, and the number one chief in the tribe. So men just don't do that, men don't get examined. You talk about prostate examinations where the doctor sticks their finger up your rectum – it seems to be so intimidating. I think men avoid showing themselves as people, human beings; they want to be men. A man is strong and if he falls, he doesn't cry; when he mashes his finger, he shakes it off … He says, "That's alright, I'm a man." He won't say 'Ouch,' and he should. But that's something I'm trying to help our men with: if you get sick say, "I'm sick." Boys don't cry, which isn't true, or they don't hurt; that's not true either. But men hurt like women hurt; they get into despair like other people get into despair. They need love. The position that women put their husbands in makes them avoid coming to doctors or telling the truth about what's going on with them.

Also, I don't think men enjoy information, especially technical information. Very few men can tell you what PSA means. In Atlanta, there was a man who had some writing on a sheet of paper and was giving it out. Halfway down the page it said, "If you've read this far, come back and get a thousand dollars from me." He found these sheets laying in the streets of Atlanta by the thousands after giving them out because we just don't read. We like pictures but we don't like reading. That's one of the things that I've adopted in my church, a reading club; a men's fellowship with guys who want to educate themselves. This is the time of technology so why not get involved? I have some guys down there who don't even know what a computer is all about. We limit ourselves in study ... We don't like to read.

Discussion

Bishop Thomas Alvin Body had the fortune to consult with a urologist when he began to notice symptoms that could be related to his prostate health. Unfortunately, millions of Americans are unable to do so because of the associated costs. Health insurance is at a premium in today's society as 20.7% of African-Americans have no coverage whatsoever. This is disconcerting for the population most aggressively targeted by certain deadly diseases (including prostate cancer) as the fraction of uninsured American has grown to 15.8%.

We have already learned through this book that the most effective way to combat prostate cancer is early detection. Keeping this in mind, refusing to seek care when experiencing symptoms can be a very deadly choice. Reverend Body effectively framed the manly man's mindset: "Boys don't cry." When a man's responsibility is to provide for his household, the financial decision between providing that care for his family and seeking care for his own health problems tends to lead him to simply, 'suck it up.' Many organizations recognize this dilemma that many families experience on a daily basis, and have begun to combat the problem.

Facts

- Studies have shown that higher socioeconomic status comes along with an increased incidence of prostate cancer; however, the incidence of death from prostate cancer is higher at lower socioeconomic status. **See charts below:**

	All		Non-Hispanic White		African-American	
SES	n	Rate	n	Rate	n	Rate
Q1	1,305	33.5	559	33.1	355	67.6
Q2	1,844	32.5	1,254	32.6	154	64.8
Q3	2,001	31	1,576	31.4	176	64.7
Q4	1,975	29.6	1,635	29.9	134	72.5
Q5	1,872	29.5	1,664	30.7	63	73.5

Quality of life effects on prostate cancer incidence in Non-Hispanic Whites and African-Americans compared to the overall population.

	All		Hispanic		Asian/Pacific Islander	
SES	n	Rate	n	Rate	n	Rate
Q1	1,305	33.5	338	27.3	53	13.9
Q2	1,844	32.5	243	27.1	93	19.3
Q3	2,001	31	177	27.9	72	15.1
Q4	1,975	29.6	123	27.9	83	15.9
Q5	1,872	29.5	72	27.8	73	14

Quality of life effects on prostate cancer incidence in Hispanics and Asian/Pacific Islanders compared to the overall population.

Recommendations

- Consult with the Centers for Medicare and Medicaid Services (CMS) to see if you qualify for any of their coverage options.

  - If you cannot receive health insurance due to a pre-existing condition, CMS has options for you!

- Several organizations sponsor free health screenings for all patients regardless of race or income level. Many of these events and clinics offer prostate cancer screenings (**DRE** and **PSA testing**) for men.

  - It is recommended that men have their prostate health checked annually. An annual health fair offering the service could complete the requirement.

  - Even if you cannot currently afford the care, **get screened!** It is always important for men to know the status of their prostate health just as with any other part of their bodies.

FACT:

"Prostate cancer is the second leading cause of cancer death in men."

CHAPTER 18
We have Options

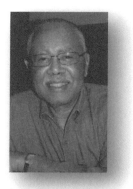

Austin Brown, Retired

I was born in Floyd County, Georgia, and later moved to Ohio when I was four years old. I'm a computer person; I've done programming system analysis and managed actual programming departments. My last job before retirement was with the DeKalb County School System where I was the assistant director of information systems and worked with student information, payroll, human resources, software and applications.

I've been a frequent visitor to doctors for a long time. My father died of a heart attack when he was 53. I'd never known him to go to a doctor, so his passing was a shock to me. I had a brother who passed away at 46. I think he died of a heart attack as well. It was either a heart attack or a stroke; I'm not sure of which one. That was a wake-up call for me since they were both heart related. I decided I would find out information, and this was before the Internet. After getting the information, I went to a doctor to see what I could do to keep myself healthy.

I believed, if my father passed away early, and my brother passed away early, the apple doesn't fall far from the tree, and I would be the same way. I found a study program in Cincinnati where they were doing a lipid study, and that was my first study from an academic standpoint. That was back in the mid-70's. My brother passed away in 1974. Coming to the Atlanta area, I got into a study with a doctor at Emory University who was doing a blood pressure study. That was back in the mid to late 80's.

My primary doctor told me I needed to get a prostate check. I was referred to Dr. Bennett. There was a study going on regarding research [that] selenium and vitamin E [might reduce the risk of developing prostate cancer]. I had been in that study since 2004. I faithfully came in to get my DRE and PSA checked every six months.

In 2009, my PSA increased to 1.5; the year before it was 0.8 or 0.7, and it was still normal. I said, "Cool, my PSA is still in the normal range, I'm not worried." Then, I get this letter saying that you've got to come in to get a biopsy. Why? I'm normal. I came in and said, "You sure I need to get a biopsy?" They explained, I needed the biopsy because it had gone up more than it was supposed to. We scheduled the biopsy and sure enough, they found prostate cancer; small, localized and slow growing.

When I got the results, I knew it was bad news because when I came into the office to see the doctor, he was already in the room; it wasn't a good sign. I was still in denial. I don't recall anything after that. My only recollection is that I forgot everything. I was reading something and it was like it was there, but it wasn't there. My wife said, "You're not answering the questions?" She made some comment, and I wasn't there in body; it's like I had gone off somewhere else. And that was the only emotional feeling that I had. I was in denial. I heard it, but I kind of like went off somewhere. My thought was, "What's he talking about?" I didn't want to believe what I was hearing, so I kind of removed myself from my surroundings. I went up on the bookshelf and I sat for a while, watched what was going on; I really wasn't there. My wife commented that Dr. Bennett had said something and that I didn't respond to him. It was almost like I insulted him, and I don't remember what it was. My wife finally said, "What are you talking about?," and so, I came back down from the bookshelf. It sounds corny; I came back into my body and said, "Okay, this is real. This is reality."

Analytically, I decided what outcome I wanted, and that was success and removal of this disease from my body. And, how was I gonna get there? That's where the spreadsheet came in. Did I want the pellets, surgery or chemo? I really didn't want any of those options although they were there for me. Therefore, I considered another research study. The good thing about the study was that if the study didn't work, I still had the other options. It was a win-win. I couldn't lose anything by trying it. If it worked, I'm cancer free, and if it didn't work, I still had the pellets [radiation therapy], the chemo[therapy], the surgery, the cryo[therapy] and all the other types of treatment that are available. Fortunately, I didn't have to go through all those drastic steps because the study treatment was successful.

I got all of the information and options from Dr. Bennett. My wife got on the computer and she started looking up stuff, and I had this book I was reading. I made a spreadsheet of all the options, questions and the answers. and I said, "I'm going to do this methodically and figure out which is the best approach for me." It took a little while to put it together. Dr. Bennett said that the study he wanted me to participate in was the WST11* study; the study where they did the injection and the little wire things that they used to zap it.

---

*WST11 references the drug used in the first multi-center prospective Prostate Cancer focal therapy trial conducted in the U.S. If you would like more information on the trial, please visit www.clinicaltrials.gov.

Let's go back to the mid 70's, when I first participated in the study of lipids in Ohio. Why do I participate in studies? Because, I need to leave a footprint on this earth that will help someone who potentially has a problem that can be fixed. If I can be a part of that group, then that's my calling, that's my responsibility. I'm not responsible for all the Black men, but for a small number in making sure that the health that we have and the treatments that we have are made available to us. If being in a study group furthers that, that's what I'll do. It's never an inconvenience to me to be in a study group. It's a privilege to be in a study group.

If more Black men would put their pride in their pocket and go see a doctor, we would have more Black men living longer lives today. To have someone say, "I don't wanna know," is like putting your head in the sand and that does other things to you; it leaves other parts of you exposed. I hurt over here in my stomach, but I'm not gonna go see a doctor because I don't wanna know. I think it's bad, but I don't wanna know. Yeah you do; you really do want to know because you want to be able to get that part fixed.

Black men are macho, proud and all of that. We don't go to see doctors. We have to get past that. We need to see a doctor who is a staunch supporter of Black men's health. It certainly helped me. Had I not been in the study group, I would probably not had access to the WST11 study. I was fortunate enough to be there a bit longer on the previous study which led into this one

Today, I am most grateful because I can wake up each morning without the threat of cancer hanging over me to be cured and not counting my days to my demise. My life is in God's hands. I'm grateful to be able to wake up each morning and be with my wife and my family and function with minimum discomfort. To see my beautiful granddaughter, is special to me. Perhaps, this is something I would not have experienced had I not been treated.

The Wife's Perspective

First, I am a wife and mother. I say this from a wife and mother's perspective; if we aren't proactive in getting out and doing the things we need to do for ourselves, then we can't expect our men to do anything either. I know a great many women who don't take care of themselves; therefore, they end up being sick with all these disease[s]. I've always been mindful of the value of good health. I come from a family of believers. As a wife and mother, I go online and search for information about health issues and then place them before my husband and sons.

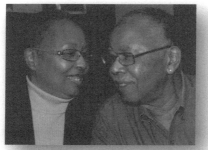

Phyllis and Austin Brown

Then, I go back and ask them, "what do you think about the information and what do you plan to do?" After a few days, I simply call the doctor, make an appointment, get them in the car and take them – period. We will soon celebrate our fiftieth anniversary, and we have travelled all over the world. This would not be possible if we did not take care of our health. We would not be here to celebrate and appreciate our first granddaughter, Elena.

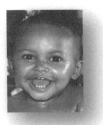

Elena, Mr. and Mr. Brown's Granddaughter

Discussion

According to the American Cancer Society, many advances in life expectancy and quality of life for cancer patients and survivors are the direct results of clinical research trials. Unfortunately, despite the tremendous potential that clinical research trials can afford to the African-American community, Mr. Austin Brown is one of only 2% of African-Americans today that participate in clinical research trials. Not only are African-Americans under-represented in clinical trials, but they are also less likely to participate in clinical trials than their Caucasian counterparts. This underrepresentation may continue to widen the gap in health disparities as results gathered from clinical research trials (CRTs) are often generalized to the entire population, despite documented genetic and racial differences making race-specific trials even more crucial.

CRTs are studies performed with patients to discover whether promising approaches to disease prevention, diagnosis and treatment are safe and effective. In order for the U.S. Food and Drug Administration (FDA) to approve a new drug or treatment, it must successfully complete three phases of clinical trials. If approved, the drug can eventually become widely available to patients and become the standard for treatment.

African-Americans are losing out on valuable research and suffering from preventable barriers in health because of fear and mistrust. Between the years of 1932 and 1972, the Tuskegee syphilis study was conducted in Tuskegee, Alabama by the U.S. Public Health Service to study the natural progression of untreated syphilis in poor, rural black men who thought they were receiving free health care from the U.S. government.[1] Lifesaving drugs were deliberately withheld to ensure that the "natural" course of the disease would be observed. The experiment was shut down after a leak to the media in 1972. Many African-American's to this day, who are aware of the study, cite that this is among the many unsatisfactory interactions that reinforce and magnify their mistrust towards the medical community.

Despite this, Mr. Brown felt and continues to feel that there are physicians in the medical community such as Dr. Bennett who have his best interest in mind. As a result, he and his wife took it upon themselves to not only do their research, but weigh their options and decided that the clinical research trial offered them more options than current medical treatment could offer.

CRTs can offer interested patients the opportunity to receive the most advanced treatment available for their particular disease condition. Participants also have the opportunity to contribute to the medical community and assist other patients who may benefit from information gained from the research trial. Mr. Brown felt responsible for not only his health but for the health of those today and tomorrow.

This is not to say clinical trials do not have their share of risks. Side effects and potential benefits differ according to the individual and the particular study. Nevertheless, that is where the power of research and self-advocacy come in. Be your own advocate! If you don't have access to perform your own research, speak with a physician with whom you trust.

Facts

- Lack of minority representation in clinical trials may perpetuate health disparities.

- African-Americans represent only 2% of those that participate in clinical research trials.

Recommendations

- Consider a clinical research trial if the current treatments present for your condition do not appeal to you.

- Visit **www.clinicaltrials.gov** for more information regarding a clinical trial near you.
- Do not enroll in a clinical trial blindly without getting all your questions answered.

- Ask questions.

- Be informed.

- If you do enroll in a clinical research trial, stay in communication with your doctor, the study staff and voice your concerns.

Medical References

Harris Y, Gorelick PB, Samuels P, Bempong I, et al. Why African Americans may not be participating in clinical trials. J Natl Med Assoc. 1996;88(10):630–634.

Participation in Cancer Clinical Trials: Race-, Sex-, and Age-Based Disparities. Vivek H. Murthy, MD, MBA; Harlan M. Krumholz, MD, SM; Cary P. Gross, MD JAMA. 2004; 291(22): 2720-2726.

Midtown Urology Prostate Screening Statement

A travesty of tremendous proportions has been potentially visited on a significant segment of our society pursuant to the recent position espoused by one of our nation's leading experts, the U.S. Preventative Services Task Force (USPSTF), regarding prostate cancer screening. The USPSTF recently released new guidelines recommending men to no longer receive prostate-specific antigen tests as part of their routine screening.

Their recommendations state that there is insufficient evidence to assess if men younger than age 75 years should be screened and patients should also defer screening unless they "have symptoms that are highly suspicious of prostate cancer." The USPSTF's simplified position would have one to believe that the worst thing about prostate cancer is being subjected to PSA screening and early detection. The USPSTF's statement also disregards common knowledge that many urologists, oncologists and prostate cancer medical experts recognize that once a patient begins to experience symptoms from the disease, there is an increased risk that the cancer would have spread beyond the prostate leaving the patient with few options for treatment. This is the exact reason that the PSA test has been utilized for early detection of cancer before symptoms appear – to offer men a chance and a choice.

The USPSTF guidelines discourage routine screenings and encourage a discussion within the patient-physician relationship as a more practical and viable substitute. How can there be such disregard and support of ignorance for a disease that is the second leading cause of cancer deaths in America? The USPSTF position is not only wrong but irresponsible. Even more disheartening is the panel's decision, which has the potential to change the face of prostate cancer diagnosis and mortality in this country, did not include an opinion of a urologist, a medical oncologist or prostate cancer survivors.

The new recommendations could undermine advances in detecting and treating prostate cancer early. Instead of moving forward, we are moving ten steps in the opposite direction. As urologists and surgeons, we are baffled that prostate cancer has been selected as the disease that healthcare providers are discouraged from doing due diligence and using available resources and tests that could detect it. The USPSTF supports its position by using controversial studies that do not show survival benefit with screening while conveniently ignoring other studies that do; in fact, show a survival advantage. There's a plethora of diseases for which we utilize interventional therapies routinely without proven survival benefit. As American-trained physicians, we are taught to identify diseases in our patients and not to ignore them. As stated in the Hippocratic Oath, physicians strive to "prevent disease whenever [we] can for prevention is preferable to cure."

The basis of the prostate screening controversy is entirely linked to the patient's right to know. We all agree that the PSA test and the Digital Rectal Exam are not the "crème de la crème" in the diagnosis of prostate cancer, but they are the best we have. The premise of the USPSTF to turn a blind eye by discouraging patients' knowledge is eerily tangential to past experiments in the medical community — The Tuskegee Experiment. Essentially, both platforms fail to acknowledge ethical issues. We know that denying a population's basic right of knowledge erodes its faith in the healthcare delivery system. For those of us who have tirelessly worked over the past two decades to level the playing field regarding access, education and the right to know, the U.S. Preventative Services Task Force's position is unconscionable. Men, in general, are far less likely to follow through on doctors' appointments. With the recently announced USPSTF guidelines, this provides men further justification to avoid seeking basic medical care.

Despite their increased risk for diagnosis and death from prostate cancer, the USPSTF also proposes no potential benefits for screening in older men, African-American men and men with a family history of prostate cancer. **We strongly disagree.** The key to the successful treatment of any cancer is early detection. And to get that early diagnosis, patients must do their due diligence and healthcare providers must do theirs.

Midtown Urology therefore, **supports** the mission of promoting and raising awareness of the importance of early detection and prevention concerning health issues for men, for prostate cancer among African-American men and men worldwide. It endorses the American Urologic Association's best practice statement, as well as the position of the National Medical Association on prostate cancer early detection which includes:

1. Initial PSA testing at 40 years
2. Both DRE and PSA as part of screening
3. An informed decision-making process
4. A multifactorial assessment of risk based on age, ethnicity, family history, PSA kinetics and density

It is our hope is that the stories that are contained in this book will not discourage you, but encourage you to **know your status and know your numbers**.

"Knowledge is power." And with screening, detection and education, knowledge is also life.

James K. Bennett, M.D., F.A.C.S. Jenelle Foote, M.D., F.A.C.S.
CEO of Midtown Urology   VP of Midtown Urology

Paul Alphonse Jr., M.D., F.A.C.S.
Partner of Midtown Urology

FACT:

"One in six men will get prostate cancer during his lifetime. However, as most prostate cancer is found early, the five-year survival rate is 99 percent."

Glossary

Absorbent Products: Pads and garments, disposable or reusable, worn to absorb leaked urine. Absorbent products include shields, undergarment pads, combination pad-pant systems, diaper-like garments and bed pads.

Anemia: A condition in which the blood is deficient in red blood cells, in haemoglobin or in total volume.

Anxiety: A debilitating condition of fear which interferes with normal life functions.

Artificial Sphincter: Sometimes complicated cases of incontinence require implantation of a device known as an artificial urinary sphincter. People who might benefit from this treatment include those who are incontinent after surgery for prostate cancer or stress incontinence, trauma victims and people with congenital defects in the urinary system. The artificial sphincter has three components including a pump, balloon reservoir and a cuff that encircles the urethra and prevents urine from leaking out. The cuff is connected to the pump which is surgically implanted in the scrotum (in men) or labia (in women). The pump can be activated (usually by squeezing or pressing a button) to deflate the cuff and permit the bladder to empty. After a brief interval, the cuff refills itself and the urethra is again closed. Because the artificial sphincter is an implant, it is subject to the risks common to implants such as infection, erosion (breaking down of tissue) and mechanical malfunction. Yet with appropriate pre-surgical evaluation, operative techniques and postoperative follow-up, many problems can be avoided and incontinent patients can experience an improved quality of life with this device.

Assisted Reproductive Technologies (ART): The new forms of fertility treatment incorporate many methods of sperm retrieval and preparation. Once the sperm have been processed to ensure optimal fertilizing potential, they are used in a variety of procedures that aid the process of conception. These procedures include artificial insemination (AI), in vitro fertilization (IVF) and sperm microinjection techniques.

Autologous: Derived from the same individual.

Behavioral Techniques: Different methods to help "retrain" the bladder and get rid of the urgency to urinate. (See biofeedback, bladder training, electrical stimulation, habit training, pelvic muscle exercises and prompted voiding).

Benign Prostatic Hyperplasia: A condition in which the prostate becomes enlarged as part of the aging process.

Benign Tumor: A tumor that is not cancerous.

Bilateral: A term describing a condition that affects both sides of the body and two paired organs such as kidneys.

Biofeedback: A procedure that uses electrodes to help people gain awareness and control of their pelvic muscles.

Bladder: A hollow muscular balloon-shaped organ that stores urine until it is excreted from the body.

Bladder Training: A behavioral technique that teaches the patient to resist or inhibit the urge to urinate, and to urinate according to a schedule rather than urinating at the urge.

Brachytherapy: Involves the placement of tiny radioactive pellets into the prostate gland. By utilizing ultrasound to place the seed pellets, damage to surrounding tissues is minimized. Approximately 13,500-16,000 rads of radiation energy is delivered directly to the prostate. This procedure is performed on an outpatient basis. It is a one-time procedure with very effective results. The 10-year follow-up outcome data parallels that of radical prostatectomy.

Cancer: The uncontrolled growth of abnormal cells in the body. Cancerous cells are also called malignant cells.

Catheter: A tube passed through the body for draining fluids or injecting them into body cavities. It may be made of elastic, elastic web, rubber, glass, metal or plastic.

Catheterization: Insertion of a slender tube through the urethra or through the anterior abdominal wall into the bladder, urinary reservoir or urinary conduit to allow urine drainage.

Chancre: A hard, syphilitic primary ulcer, the first sign of syphilis, appears approximately two to three weeks after infection. The ulcer begins as a painless lesion or papule that ulcerates. Occurs generally singly, but sometimes may be multiple.

Chemolysis: Certain types of kidney stones can be dissolved with the application of chemicals. Uric acid stones, for example, can be dissolved with a solution of sodium bicarbonate in saline. Cystine stones may be treated successfully with a combination of acetylcysteine and sodium bicarbonate in saline. Struvite and carbon apatite stones can be treated with an acidic solution of hemiacidrin. The procedure involves infusing the chemical solution into the affected area by means of a ureteral catheter in a series of treatments over time until the stone is dissolved. The patient's urine must be cultured regularly throughout the course of treatment to guard against urinary infection and prevent the build up of excessive chemical levels, particularly magnesium, which can cause other health problems.

Colon: The large intestine.

Creatinine: A waste product that is filtered from the blood by the kidneys and expelled in urine.

Cryotherapy: During an operation, probes are placed in the prostate. The probes are then frozen which kills the prostatic cells.

Cyst: A lump filled with either fluid or soft material occurring in any organ or tissue; may occur for a number of reasons but is usually harmless unless its presence disrupts organ or tissue function.

Cystocele: A herniation of bladder into vagina.

Cystectomy: Surgical removal of the bladder.

Cystoscopy: A flexible scope is inserted into the urethra and then into the bladder to determine abnormalities in the bladder and lower urinary tract.

Diabetes Mellitus: A common form of diabetes in which the body cannot properly store or use glucose (sugar); the body's main source of energy.

Diuretic: A drug that increases the amount of water in the urine, removing excess water from the body; used in treating high blood pressure and fluid retention.

Electrohydraulic Lithotripsy (EHL): This technique uses a special probe to break up small stones with shock waves generated by electricity. Through a flexible ureteroscope, the physician positions the tip of the Probe 1 mm from the stone. Then, by means of a foot switch, the physician projects electrically generated hydraulic shock waves through an irrigating fluid at the stone until it is broken into small fragments. These can be passed by the patient or removed through the previously described extraction methods. EHL has some limitations: It requires general anesthesia, and is generally not used in close proximity to the kidney itself as the shock waves can cause tissue damage. Fragments produced by the hydraulic shock also tend to scatter widely, making retrieval or extraction more difficult.

Enterocele: Herniation of small bowel into vagina.

Estrogen: Hormones responsible for the development of female sex characteristics; produced by the ovary.

External Beam Radiation Therapy: A 25-28 treatment protocol that utilizes External Beam Radiation. Approximately 6800-7400 rads of radiation energy is delivered to the prostate. There can be some radiation effect on surrounding tissues.

Extracorporeal Shock Wave Lithotripsy (ESWL): Extracorporeal shock wave lithotripsy uses highly focused impulses projected from outside the body to pulverize kidney stones.

Fistula: An abnormal opening between two organs that should not be connected.

Habit Training: A behavioral technique that calls for scheduled toileting at regular intervals on a planned basis. Unlike bladder training, there is no systematic effort to motivate the patient to delay voiding and resist urge.

Hormonal Therapy: Involves the use of anti-androgens. An androgen is a male hormone needed for the production of testosterone. By depriving the cancer cells of the testosterone they need for growth, tumors regress in size and cellular activity. Side effects include gynecomastia, the enlargement of breast tissue, hot flashes and loss of libido (desire to have sex). Some long-term hormonal therapy is associated with the loss of muscle mass, osteoporosis and malaise (loss of energy).

Hydrocele: A painless swelling of the scrotum caused by a collection of fluid around the testicle; commonly occurs in middle-aged men.

Hypermobility: A condition in which the pelvic floor muscles can no longer provide the necessary support to the urethra and bladder neck. As a result, the bladder neck drops when any downward pressure is applied and causes involuntary leakage. This condition is the most common cause of stress urinary incontinence.

Hyperplasia: Excessive growth of normal cells of an organ.

Impotence: The partial or total loss of an erection which can be caused by a variety of prostate-cancer treatments or by older age. The condition may be temporary or permanent. Regardless of the cause, it can be treated by medication, a vacuum device or the injection of a drug into the penis to increase blood flow to the organ.

Incontinence: The partial or total loss of urinary control that can occur from a variety of prostate-cancer treatments or from advanced age. Incontinence can be treated with an artificial sphincter or by collagen injections.

Insemination: The placement of semen into a woman's uterus, cervix or vagina.

InterStim Continence Control Therapy: A therapy used in treating urge incontinence. Devices about the size of a pacemaker which is implanted into the sacral nerves of the lower spine where it delivers electrical impulses that help regulate bladder function.

Interstitial Laser: A laser probe is placed within prostatic tissue. Laser energy is then used to destroy prostatic tissue which makes urination easier.

Intrinsic Sphincter Deficiency (ISD): Weakening of the urethra sphincter muscles. As a result of this weakening, the sphincter does not function normally regardless of the position of the bladder neck or urethra. This condition is a common cause of stress urinary incontinence.

Irritable Bladder: Involuntary contractions of muscles in the bladder which can cause lack of control of urination.

Kegel Exercises: Exercises to strengthen the muscles of the pelvic floor which leads to more control and prevents leakage.

Kidney: One of a pair of organs located at the back of the abdominal cavity. Kidneys make urine through blood filtration.

Kidney Stone: A hard mass composed of substances from the urine that form in the kidneys.

Laparoscopic Lymph Node Dissection: If a perineal prostatectomy is contemplated prior to the operation, the pelvic lymph nodes are sampled via three small incisions made in the abdomen, much like the procedure used to remove gallbladders.

Laparoscopy: Surgery using a laparoscope to visualize internal organ through a small incision. Generally less invasive than traditional surgeries. Requires a shorter recovery period.

Lithotripsy: A procedure done to break up stones in the urinary tract using ultrasonic shock waves so that the fragments can be easily passed from the body.

Menopause: The period that marks the permanent cessation of menstrual activity usually occurring between the ages of 40 and 58.

Metastasis: The spreading of a cancerous tumor to another part of the body.

Microwave (Targis): A catheter is placed within the bladder and positioned within the prostate, then the antenna emits microwaves. This procedure increases the passageway allowing for easier urination.

Mixed Incontinence: Having both stress and urge incontinence.

Nephrectomy: Removal of an entire kidney.

Open Nephrolithotomy: Is the most invasive procedure for removing kidney stones. Because it is so traumatic, most kidneys can withstand no more than two such operations. Deep anesthesia is required after which the surgeon makes a large (10-20 centimeter) incision in the patient's back or abdomen, depending upon where the stone is located. Either the ureter or the kidney is opened and the stone extracted. Most patients require prolonged hospitalization afterward, and recovery may take up to two months.

Orchiectomy: The surgical removal of one or both of the testicles.

Orchitis: Inflammation of a testicle.

Overactive bladder: A condition characterized by involuntary bladder muscle contractions which the patient cannot suppress during the bladder filling phase.

Overflow UI: Leakage of small amounts of urine from a bladder that is always full.

Pelvic Muscle Exercises: Pelvic muscle exercises are intended to improve your pelvic muscle tone and prevent leakage for sufferers of Stress Urinary Incontinence. Also, called Kegel exercises. (See biofeedback.)

Percutaneous Nephrolithotomy (PCN): Percutaneous means "though the skin." In PCN, the surgeon or urologist makes a 1-centimeter incision under local anesthesia in the patient's back, through which an instrument called a nephroscope is passed directly into the kidney and, if necessary, the ureter. Smaller stones may be manually extracted. Large ones may need to be broken up with ultrasonic, electrohydraulic or laser- tipped probes before they can be extracted. A tube may be inserted into the kidney for drainage.

Periurethral bulking injections: A surgical procedure in which injected implants are used to "bulk up" the area around the neck of the bladder; allowing it to resist increases in abdominal pressure which can push down on the bladder and cause leakage.

Post-void Residual (PVR) Volume: A diagnostic test which measures how much urine remains in the bladder after urination. Specific measurement of PVR volume can be accomplished by catheterization, pelvic ultrasound, radiography or radioisotope studies.

Prostaglandin: Any of various oxygenated unsaturated cyclic fatty acids of animals that have a variety of hormone like actions (as in controlling blood pressure or smooth muscle contraction).

Prostate: A muscular, walnut-sized gland that surrounds part of the urethra. It secretes seminal fluid, a milky substance that combines with sperm (produced in the testicles) to form semen.

Prostatectomy: Surgical removal of the prostate.

Perineal Prostatectomy: A perineal incision is utilized. The advantages are: less blood loss, easier visualization of the bladder/urethral anastomosis and decreased recovery time because the incision does not involve muscle or any other vital tissue.

Radical Retropubic Prostatectomy: Removal of prostate through an abdominal incision. The prostate is completely removed. The advantage is that the lymph nodes can be sampled at the time of the operation and the nerve-sparing procedure is easier to do via this operation.

Suprapubic/Retropubic Prostatectomy: This involves the removal of obstructing prostatic tissue through a supra-pubic incision (a cut below the belly button). The Prostate is not wholly removed.

Suprapubic Prostatectomy requires incising the bladder to remove the obstructing tissue while a **retropubic** approach involves incising the prostatic capsule to remove the obstructing tissue. Both approaches utilize an abdominal incision.

Prostatic Stent: Inserted through a cystoscope, it is a wire device that expands after placement, thus pushing prostate tissue away from the passageway allowing for easier urination.

Prostatitis: Inflammation of the prostate.

Prostatron: Also called TUMT or Transurethral Microwave Thermotherapy. A catheter is placed within the bladder and positioned within the prostate, and then the antenna emits microwaves. This procedure increases the passageway allowing for easier urination.

Pubovaginal Sling: A surgical procedure in which a man-made or cadaveric piece of material is placed under the bladder neck to support and immobilize. This technique improves sphincter function and decreases bladder neck movement, improving continence.

Pyelonephritis: Inflammation of the kidney usually due to a bacterial infection.

Pyuria: The presence of pus in the urine; usually an indication of kidney or urinary tract infection.

Rectocele: A herniation of rectum into vagina.

Sexually Transmitted Disease (STD): Infections that are most commonly spread through sexual intercourse or genital contact.

Sling Procedures: Surgical methods for treating urinary incontinence involving the placement of a sling made either of tissue obtained from the person undergoing the sling procedure or a synthetic material. The sling is anchored to retropubic and/or abdominal structures.

Sphincter: A ring of muscle fibers located around an opening in the body that regulates the passage of substances.

Stress Test: A diagnostic test that requires patients to lift something or perform an exercise to determine if there is urine loss when stress is placed on bladder muscles.

Stress Urinary Incontinence: Urinary Incontinence: The involuntary loss of urine during period of increased abdominal pressure. Such events include laughing, sneezing, coughing or lifting heavy objects.

Testosterone: The sex hormone that stimulates development of male sex characteristics and bone and muscle growth; produced by the testicles and in small amounts by the ovaries.

Transient Urinary Incontinence: Temporary episodes of urinary incontinence that is gone when the cause of the episode is identified and treated.

Resources

American Cancer Society
250 Williams St. NW, #6000
Atlanta, GA 30303
Phone: 1-800-227-2345
Web Address: www.cancer.org

The American Cancer Society is a nationwide community-based voluntary health organization dedicated to eliminating cancer as a major health problem. Headquartered in Atlanta, Georgia, the ACS has 12 chartered divisions, more than 900 local offices nationwide, and a presence in more than 5,100 communities.

American Prostate Society
1340-F Charwood Rd.
Hanover, MD 21076
Phone: 410-859-3735
Web Address: www.ameripros.org

A leading blog dedicated to prostate health, management and prevention. This blog also offers other valuable resources for more information.

Cancer Care, Inc.
275 7th Avenue
New York, NY 10001
Phone: 800-813-4673
 212-712-8400
Web Address: www.cancercare.org

Cancer Care was founded with the mission of helping advanced cancer patients. This is done through counseling, support groups, and professional information and support.

Cancer Support Community
1050 17th St NW, Suite 500
Washington, DC 20036

Phone: 1-888-793-9355
202-659-9709
Web Address: www.cancersupportcommunity.org

An international non-profit concerned with supporting, educating and giving hope to men with cancer. A large employer of psychosocial oncology mental health professionals in the United States.

Centers for Disease Control and Prevention (CDC)
1600 Clifton Road
Atlanta, GA 30333
Phone: 1-800-232-4636
404-639-3534
Web Address: www.cdc.gov

CDC has been dedicated to protecting health and promoting quality of life through the prevention and control of disease, injury and disability. The organization is committed to programs that reduce the health and economic consequences of the leading causes of death and disability; thereby, ensuring a long, productive and healthy life for all people.

Dattoli Cancer Foundation
2803 Fruitville Road
Sarasota, FL 34237
Phone: 1-800-915-1001
941-365-5599
Web Address: www.dattolifoundation.org

A nonprofit cancer foundation that provides prostate cancer information, support and literature to men with prostate cancer. Provides resources and guidance for men dealing with a prostate cancer diagnosis.

Department of Veterans Affairs
810 Vermont Ave. NW
Washington, DC 20420

Phone: 1-800-827-1000
                202-273-5400
Web Address: www.va.gov

The department of Veterans Affairs aims to fulfill President Lincoln's promise to serve and honor the men and women who are America's veterans.

Georgia Prostate Cancer Coalition
5588 Chamblee-Dunwoody Road #150
Dunwoody, GA 30338
Phone: 404-448-3127
Web Address: www.georgiapcc.org

The Georgia Prostate Cancer Coalition, Inc. is a non-profit (501c3) organization founded by representatives from various prostate cancer support groups in the Metro-Atlanta area. Georgia Prostate Cancer Coalition is a coalition partner with the National Prostate Cancer Coalition (NPCC) and a member of the National Alliance of State Prostate Cancer Coalitions. The mission is to increase prostate cancer awareness, advocacy and information exchange.

Health Insurance Association of America (HIAA)
555 13th St. NW. Ste. 600
East Washington, D.C. 20004
Phone: 202-824-1600
Web Address: www.hiaa.org

Offers and advocates for expanding access to affordable health coverage to all Americans.

HIS PROSTATE CANCER
Web Address: www.hisprostatecancer.com

The website was created to help you during this difficult time. It provides information to support you and your loved one as you make important decisions such as choosing among the many treatment options.

Male Care: Men Fighting Cancer, Together
Web Address: www.malecare.org

America's largest volunteer men's cancer support group and advocacy national nonprofit organization. America's first and leading gay men's cancer survivor national nonprofit.

Midtown Urology Health and Education Foundation (MUHEF)
128 North Avenue
Atlanta, GA 30308
Phone: 404-881-0966
Web Address: www.midtown-urology.com

MUHEF is a nonprofit organization established to address the health disparities facing minority communities. Its mission is to foster a progressive interest in the overall health of the medically underserved in the Atlanta metropolitan area and the state of Georgia by facilitating educational seminars, health screenings, peer counseling and clinical research development. To carry out this mission, it hosts a series of community service programs.

National Association for Continence (NAFC)
P.O Box 1019
Charleston, SC 29402
Phone: 1-800-BLADDER (1-800-252-3337)
Web Address: www.nafc.org

NAFC is a nonprofit national organization with a mission of consumer advocacy, education of the public, and information dissemination through collaboration and networking for the benefit of those with urinary incontinence. NAFC's booklet, "Your Personal Guide to Bladder Health" can be ordered on the NAFC web site.

National Kidney and Urologic Diseases Information Clearinghouse (NKUDIC)
3 Information Way
Bethesda, MD 20892
Phone: 1-800-891-5390
Web Address: www.kidney.niddk.nih.gov

The NKUDIC, a federal agency, is a service of the National Institute of Diabetes and Digestive and Kidney Diseases (NIDDK). NIDDK is part of the National Institutes of Health under the U.S. Department of Health and Human Services. The clearinghouse provides information about diseases of the kidneys and urologic system to people with kidney and urologic disorders and to their families, health professionals and the public. NKUDIC answers inquiries; develops, reviews and distributes publications and works closely with professional and patient groups and government agencies to coordinate resources about kidney and urologic diseases.

Prost Aware
Web address: www.prostaware.org

Prost Aware is the greater Atlanta area's prostate cancer awareness resource for men and their loved ones. Prost Aware takes an unique cancer awareness approach by raising awareness through music and technology.

The Prostate Conditions Education Council
7009 S. Potomac Street, #125
Centennial, CO 80112
Web Address: www.pcaw.org

The Prostate Conditions Education Council (PCEC) was founded in 1989, and is a non-profit 501-3c organization. The Council is comprised of a consortium of leading physicians, health educators, scientists and prostate cancer advocates.

Prostate Cancer Foundation (PCF)
1250 Fourth St.
Santa Monica, CA 90401
Phone: 1-800-757-CURE (1-877-757-2873)
310-570-4700
Web Address: www.pcf.org

The leading philanthropic organization funding and accelerating prostate cancer research globally.

Social Security Administration
Windsor Park Bldg.
Office of Public Inquiries
6401 Security Blvd.
Baltimore, MD 21235
Phone: 1-800-772-1213
Web Address: www.ssa.gov

The Social Security Administration is in place to provide retirement and disability benefits among other types of benefits.

Urology Health.org, American Urological Association
1000 Corporate Blvd.
Linthicum, MD 21090
Phone: 1-800-828-7866
410-689-3700
Web Address: www.urologyhealth.org

UrologyHealth.org is a website written by urologists for patients. Visitors can find specific topics by using the "search" option. The web site provides information about adult and pediatric urologic topics including kidney, bladder, and prostate conditions. You can find a urologist, sign up for a free quarterly newsletter or click on the Urology Resource Center to find materials about urologic problems.

US TOO International Prostate Cancer Education and Support Network (Us TOO)
5003 Fairview Ave.
Downers Grove, IL 60515
Phone: 630-795-1002
Web Address: **www.ustoo.org**

A nonprofit prostate cancer education and support network that provides men and their families with information and support to make informed decisions regarding prostate detection, treatment and surviving.

You Are Not Alone Now (YANA): Prostate Cancer Support Site
Web Address: **www.yananow.org**

A support site dedicated to providing any man diagnosed with prostate cancer with information to guide them in making the right decisions for themselves in the areas of diagnosis and treatment.

ZERO: The Project to End Prostate Cancer
10 G St. NE, Suite 601
Washington, DC 20002
Phone: 202-463-9455
Web Address: **www.zerocancer.org**

The ultimate goal is to create a life-giving legacy for our sons and grandsons: the first generation of men who are free from prostate cancer – "Generation ZERO."